# *H*olistic
# Pregnancy
## *and* Childbirth

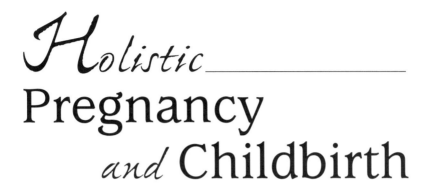

# Holistic Pregnancy and Childbirth

JAMES MARTI

*with* Heather Burton

John Wiley & Sons, Inc.

New York    Chichester    Weinheim    Brisbane    Singapore    Toronto

Published by John Wiley & Sons, Inc.
Published simultaneously in Canada.

Design and production by Navta Associates, Inc.

The information contained in this book is not intended to serve as a replacement for professional medical advice. Any use of the information in this book is at the reader's discretion. The author and publisher specifically disclaim any and all liability arising directly or indirectly from the use or application of any information contained in this book. A health care professional should be consulted regarding your specific situation.

*Library of Congress Cataloging-in-Publication Data:*

Marti, James
  Holistic pregnancy and childbirth / James Marti, with Heather Burton.
     p.    cm.
  Includes index.
  ISBN 0-471-18509-4 (paper : alk. paper)
    1. Pregnancy—Popular works.   2. Childbirth—Popular works.   3. Holistic medicine.
  I. Burton, Heather.   II. Title.
  RG525.M3337   1999
  618.2'4—dc21                                          98-27943
Printed in the United States of America

10  9  8  7  6  5  4  3  2  1

This book is dedicated to Beth Molesworth,
who twenty-three years ago led the way—
giving birth to a beautiful boy
and, without knowing it, to this book.

# CONTENTS

# $\mathcal{A}$CKNOWLEDGMENTS

MORE THAN THREE YEARS went into the preparation of this book. I am personally indebted to Heather Burton, founder of the Midwifery Alliance, for sharing her considerable knowledge of holistic therapy. Her careful research and meticulous editing and writing made this book possible, and her sense of humor and the materials from her childbirth classes were invaluable assets.

I am also grateful to the many health care professionals and organizations that answered queries, faxed us their guidelines, and provided insight and inspiration. Special thanks to the helpful staff at the American College of Obstetricians and Gynecologists; the American Academy of Pediatrics; the Healthy Mothers, Healthy Babies Coalition; ASPO/Lamaze; the National Association of Childbirth Centers; Informed Birth and Parenting; the International Association of Parents and Professionals for Safe Alternatives in Childbirth; the International Childbirth Education Association; La Leche League International; and the San Francisco Medical Research Foundation. Special thanks must also be given to the specialists on the Medical Advisory Board for this book, who reviewed chapters and recommended holistic therapies. I am especially indebted to Drs. John Mabrey and Abel Jimenez who reviewed the entire manuscript and answered the publisher's queries prior to publication.

I also wish to thank the staff at the University of California at San Francisco Medical Library and at the Lane Medical Library at Stanford University who patiently helped us comb through hundreds of medical journals. Head Librarian Kathy Resnick at the Marin General Hospital Library was especially helpful in conducting a Medline search for the latest holistic approaches to pregnancy and childbirth used worldwide.

Thanks to Laurie Harper, my literary agent, who is the best at what she does—combining intelligence, competence, and a wry sense of humor—and found the perfect publisher.

I am also grateful to the pioneers of holistic medicine whose work inspired this book. In the last twenty-five years, the works of Drs. Herbert Benson, Joan Borysenko, Bernie Siegel, Andrew T. Weil, Dean Ornish, and Deepak Chopra have become internationally prominent. These holistic practitioners believe passionately in the remarkable power of the body to heal itself, and this book serves as a testament to their work.

Many personal friends also contributed to this book; without their support, inspiration, and diversion, I would surely have failed. Thank you, Frankie Stream and Karen McCrystal, for your conscientious editing. Thank you, Andrea Hine, for your graciousness and unequaled gentility. Thank you, Alan Davis, for being the best friend in the world. Thanks, David Grabill, for your friendship of thirty years. Thank you, Margit Bauer, for your hospitality. Thank you, Dr. Raphael Ornstein, for giving me my early education in holistic medicine. Thanks also to Mitch Rofski, Dr. Jean Fryer, my brothers John and David Marti, my mother, and Jesse Molesworth (for showing me the essentials of clear writing). Thanks also, Edwin Treitler, publisher of *New Visions,* for our enchanting conversations and meditations.

I also wish to thank my friend and colleague, Carole Hall, Associate Publisher at Wiley, for believing in this book. I remain eternally indebted to Judith McCarthy, my editor at Wiley, for her astute and very readable corrections and suggestions. The whole team at Wiley, a very special publisher, made possible my dream.

# $\mathcal{I}$NTRODUCTION

THIS BOOK IS ABOUT A JOURNEY—a journey of love, birth, and healing; a journey as old as humanity itself. *Holistic Pregnancy and Childbirth* charts a path for those who are about to experience the miracle of childbirth.

Twenty-two years ago, when my son was born, there were no books on holistic pregnancy. Fortunately, his mother, Beth, and I were studying in Arica, a school of yoga and medication, where we learned more than fifty exercises in relaxation, breathing, massage, and intimacy. There is nothing more beautiful than watching a conscious, healthy woman give birth. Beth's daily routine during her pregnancy —a program of meditation, yoga, exercise, diet, aromatherapy, botanical medicine, homeopathy, and tai chi—was a wonder to behold, and this book is dedicated to her. I remember thinking then, and I believe it even more strongly now, that giving birth naturally and with the highest consciousness means hope for future civilization.

Like most fathers, I thought my son was the most beautiful boy the moment he was born; and for me, his birth was the most precious blessing of my life. In all the years since, there has never been a moment when I did not feel this way. Although I have never told him so (it would embarrass him, I think), he has always been my teacher and my guide, and I feel connected with the higher order of things whenever I am in his presence.

I have personally witnessed the effects of the holistic therapies and exercises included in this book, and I know that they work. The beauty of these exercises is that they may not only help you give birth to a healthy, beautiful baby, they may also enhance the parents' lives immeasurably. Mother, father, and child will become a relaxed, healthy, considerate, physically active, and emotionally bonded family.

In the last ten years, there has been a remarkable improvement in the outcome of pregnancy for mothers as well as for infants. More women enter pregnancy healthier; they get better, more complete prenatal care; and new holistic options are available for conception, pregnancy, and childbirth. This book presents important new information—not just about holistic childbirth, but also the nine months that precede it; not just about the risks that pregnancy presents, but also the many holistic approaches that minimize or eliminate these risks; and not just about the medical aspects of pregnancy, but also the psychological and emotional changes that occur. It is my sincerest hope that this book will enable you to have the most beautiful pregnancy and childbirth possible, and that you will help spread the word about holistic medicine.

Once, while my son was still growing inside his mother's womb, I asked a wise man for his advice on how to raise a child. He told me, "Raise your child to be a fool, and he will become a fool. Raise him to become a Buddha, and he'll become a Buddha!"

His advice has guided me in raising my son and also in the preparation of this book, and I fervently hope it will benefit you as well.

## Chapter 1

# The Holistic Program for Pregnancy and Childbirth

*T*HE WORD IS SPREADING. The breakthroughs in holistic medicine are announced virtually every day. The best-selling holistic medical books written by Doctors Deepak Chopra, Bernie Siegel, Dean Ornish, and Andrew Weil, as well as other practitioners, have brought holistic medicine to center stage.

A self-healing/transformation approach is at the center of holistic medicine; in fact, the leading proponents of holistic medicine use words such as "transformation" or "transcendence" to describe their approach. In *Peace, Love and Healing,* Siegel states, "We all have the ability to train our bodies to heal and eliminate illness. I think we can use meditative and lifestyle-altering techniques . . . to gain access to the superintelligence I'm convinced resides within each of us." Chopra writes, in *Perfect Health: The Complete Mind/Body Guide,* "If you live in tune with your quantum mechanical body, all of your daily activities will proceed smoothly . . . breathing, eating, digestion, assimilation, and elimination. The most important routine to follow is transcending, the act of getting in touch with the quantum level of yourself."

*Holistic Pregnancy and Childbirth* was written to help you make your pregnancy and childbirth the most beautiful experience of your life. We believe that you can use the holistic approach to have a more comfortable pregnancy, a shorter labor, and the joyful delivery of a perfectly healthy baby. From conception through the first few months after delivery, you'll feel more confident and energetic using the natural holistic methods outlined in this book. They are designed to help you sleep more soundly, nourish yourself on delicious, nutritious foods, and enjoy a wonderful sexual intimacy with your partner. And we hope that, like the women profiled in this book, you will be able to deliver your baby without drugs or surgery, unless absolutely necessary.

*Holistic Pregnancy and Childbirth* addresses the concerns you are likely to have about your baby's development; possible complications; emergencies that require intervention; diet; and methods of preventing and treating the normal pain and discomfort of pregnancy, labor, birth, and the period immediately following birth (postpartum).

Individual chapters guide you in monitoring physical changes in yourself and your baby; choosing a holistic caregiver, preparing a Holistic Birth Plan; designing an optimum meal plan and personal exercise program; practicing a daily relaxation program of yoga, visualization, meditation, and breathing exercises; deciding where you want to have your baby; choosing a method of labor and delivery that will reduce the risk of complications and the need for surgical interventions, such as a cesarean delivery (C-section) or episiotomy; adopting holistic approaches to bonding, postpartum recovery, and breastfeeding; and preventing common baby discomforts during the first precious weeks of your child's life.

In choosing the holistic approaches recommended in this book, we used the following criteria:

1. Every procedure must be holistic. Holistic medicine is mind/body medicine. It is applied as though you and your fetus constitute a single, whole organism. Pain relief during pregnancy, labor, birth, and postpartum should stimulate the body to produce its own natural painkillers—the endorphins.

2. Every procedure must be noninvasive and safe for the mother and baby. As Hippocrates once said, "Above all else, do no harm." This book does not recommend practices and procedures that are not supported by scientific evidence as necessary for a healthy pregnancy, including enemas, IV (intravenous) drips, oxytocin-induced labor, episiotomy, or cesarean deliveries; electronic fetal

monitoring is also not recommended by the authors. Although any of these procedures may be recommended in an emergency, you should make the final decision to allow their use only after your caregiver has presented clinical evidence that the procedure is necessary and safe for you and your baby.

3. Every procedure must be effective and focus on the *prevention* of discomfort and complications rather than merely the treatment of disorders once they develop. From acupuncture to yoga, every procedure recommended in this book is designed to help strengthen the immune system and prevent problems that might be caused by nutritional deficiencies or psychological or physiological stress.

The comprehensive holistic program outlined in this book is based on information compiled from four principal sources: (1) recommendations and suggestions of members of our Medical Advisory Board; (2) guidelines and recommendations of the American College of Obstetricians and Gynecologists (ACOG), the American Academy of Pediatrics, the Healthy Mothers, Healthy Babies Coalition, the American Society for Psychoprophylaxis in Obstetrics (ASPO), the National Association of Childbirth Centers, Informed Birth and Parenting, the International Association of Parents and Professionals for Safe Alternatives in Childbirth, the International Childbirth Education Association, La Leche League International, the San Francisco Medical Research Foundation, the Read Childbirth Foundation, the American Dietetic Association (ADA), and the National Association of Childbirth Assistants (NACA); (3) new clinical research on conception, pregnancy, labor, delivery, and maternal and newborn care reported in medical journals worldwide; and (4) firsthand accounts and profiles of midwives and mothers who used holistic methods during pregnancy and childbirth. References to citations, monthly checkup checklists, and organizations to contact for additional information are listed at the back of the book.

## $\mathcal{T}$YPES OF HOLISTIC THERAPIES

Holistic medicine involves many specialized procedures, each of which might be said to constitute a spoke on a medicine wheel. The combination of holistic approaches recommended in this book constitutes a program that has been clinically proven safe and effective for conception, pregnancy, labor, childbirth, and newborn care. Many of these approaches are used in different parts of the world, including India (Ayurvedic), China (traditional Chinese medicine), Greece (naturopathic), Europe (homeopathic), and the United States (allopathic). They include acupuncture and acupressure, aromatherapy, Ayurvedic medicine, Bach flower remedies, breathing techniques, botanical medicine, chiropractic, nutrition and supplements, homeopathy, hydrotherapy, hypnosis, intimacy exercises, massage, meditation, osteopathy, qigong, physical activity, traditional Chinese medicine (TCM), and yoga. An overview of these approaches follows. In appropriate chapters, you'll discover how to use each of them to have a healthy and comfortable pregnancy.

## Acupuncture and Acupressure

Acupuncture and acupressure are the most widely used holistic procedures for childbirth in the East. They originated in China more than 5,000 years ago and are used to stimulate the vital life force (called *chi*) which flows through thirteen channels (*meridians*) in the body.

Acupuncturists use needles to stimulate the meridians, which trigger the release of *endorphins*—natural substances released by nerves to relieve pain. It might seem odd to stick a pregnant woman with needles, but the needles penetrate just below the skin's surface and don't draw blood or cause any discomfort for you or your baby. Acupressure (also called shiatsu) therapists use their fingers and thumbs to stimulate chi points on the surface of the body.

Both acupuncture and acupressure have been used safely to relieve certain disorders—such as high blood pressure, digestive disorders, skin problems, fatigue, bladder and kidney problems, headaches, insomnia, nausea and vomiting, and muscle tension—even during pregnancy. Acupuncture has also been used to stimulate labor and to relieve pain while babies in the breech position are turned.

Whether you would benefit from acupuncture or acupressure depends on the severity of your symptoms and the availability of skilled practitioners in your community. Acupuncture should be performed by a licensed professional; we strongly recommend that you select a practitioner who specializes in pregnancy and childbirth. Acupressure can be self-administered, although you should first consult with a licensed therapist to identify the chi points for specific discomforts precisely. We've included the names and location of appropriate acupressure points in each chapter for illustrative purposes, only.

## Aromatherapy

You might not realize it, but we're all extremely sensitive to aromas. If we faint, for example, a whiff of smelling salts will usually quickly revive us.

Aromas have also been used during pregnancy to relieve many discomforts, including nausea, heartburn, fatigue, dizziness, and headaches. In aromatherapy, essential oils derived from the leaves, barks, roots, flowers, resins, or seeds of plants are inhaled or applied to the skin, or added to a bath for skin and muscle problems. The chemical makeup of each oil is believed to be responsible for its pharmacological properties, which include antibacterial, antiviral, antispasmodic, diuretic (promoting urine flow), vasodilatory (widening blood vessels to increase blood flow), and vasoconstrictor (narrowing blood vessels to decrease blood flow) effects.

Because inhaled aromas are transferred very quickly from the nose to the brain, they are especially effective in stimulating endorphin production and relieving anxiety and tension.

## Ayurvedic Medicine

In his book, *Quantum Healing,* Dr. Deepak Chopra describes how he cured a 39-year-old woman with lymphatic cancer by using Ayurvedic medicine. The treatment included healthy food choices, Indian herbs, massage, meditation, and yoga.

In Sanskrit, Ayurveda means "the science of life and longevity." According to Chopra, "The guiding principle of Ayurveda is that the mind exerts the deepest influence on the body, and freedom from sickness depends upon contacting our own awareness, bringing it into balance, and then extending that balance to the body. This state of balanced awareness . . . creates a higher state of health." Ayurvedic medicine uses a variety of physical and psychological therapies, including yoga, massage, aromatherapy, diet, meditation, and botanical medicine. During your pregnancy, it may help relieve morning sickness, vomiting, nausea, fatigue, flatulence, migraines, nasal congestion, vaginal infections, and backaches.

## Bach Flowers

The first healing system known to be based on flower essences was developed in 1930 by the Welsh homeopath, Edward Bach, a physician and pathologist who experimented with "the healing secrets of wildflowers" to cure himself of depression. Bach believed that certain wildflowers had subtle life energies that could heal specific emotional disorders. By the time of his death, he had invented thirty-eight remedies based on wildflowers, including honeysuckle, holly, and wild rose.

Bach flower remedies, which are taken either as tinctures (alcohol-based solutions) or in capsules, are used to relieve many of the results of stress during pregnancy, especially migraine headaches and insomnia. Midwives and naturopathic obstetricians in Canada and Britain are trained to use Bach flowers to treat pregnant women, and have reportedly used them to prevent miscarriages. Midwives now routinely recommend one Bach flower formula, Rescue Remedy, to relieve fatigue and dizziness during pregnancy and pain and discomfort during labor.

## Biofeedback

Twenty-five years ago, Western doctors developed electronic equipment called *biofeedback machines* to help patients regulate involuntary responses to stress. People suffering from migraine headaches, for example, can be connected to biofeedback machines that monitor their body temperature, blood pressure, heart rate, or brainwaves. While hooked up to a biofeedback machine, patients can be trained to consciously alter these functions; for example, to lower their blood pressure.

Biofeedback has been used during pregnancy and labor to relieve discomfort due to incontinence, postural changes, back pain, gastrointestinal disorders, and fatigue, as well as tension and migraine headaches.

## Botanical Medicine

For centuries before the advent of manufactured drugs, pregnant women throughout the world took botanical medicines, which contain plant extracts, to strengthen the immune system and relieve many of the common discomforts of pregnancy. In China, pregnant women are still not usually given prescription drugs by their caregivers, but rather packets of herbs, or botanical medicines.

All botanical medicines, teas, infusions, and poultices recommended in this book have been used safely and effectively by pregnant women. Some, like chamomile tea, have been used safely and effectively to aid digestion and relieve insomnia. Others, like nettle tea, have been used to relieve anemia, leg cramps, and kidney troubles. Fennel tea and slippery elm tea have been used to reduce indigestion and morning sickness. Mu tea is believed to help give you energy, as is Japanese bancha or kukicha tea. These teas are still routinely recommended by midwives and herbalists for pregnant women. Nevertheless, as an added precaution, you should discuss the use of any botanical remedy with your caregiver.

## Breathing

Learning how to breathe properly might seem about as necessary as learning how to scratch an itch or blink. Because we do it automatically from the day we're born, we take it for granted that we know how to breathe correctly.

Studies show, however, that most pregnant women don't always breathe as efficiently as they should. Improper breathing—especially rapid, shallow breathing (hyperventilation)—heightens your body's response to stress, thereby increasing your heart rate and blood pressure and the concentration of stress hormones (including cortisol and epinephrine [adrenaline]) in your blood. The stress response can affect the health of both you and your baby. In Chapter 4, we describe many breathing exercises designed to reduce the stress response.

Correct breathing is vital for relaxation and for increasing the amount of oxygen supplied to you and your baby. Your baby's lungs are still developing and can't get oxygen on their own until they mature (at birth). Therefore, the fetus takes oxygen from your blood as it passes through the placenta straight into its own bloodstream. By breathing correctly, you're more likely to supply your baby with as much oxygen as it needs.

Breathing exercises are also integral to meditation and autosuggestion, or self-hypnosis. They're also excellent ways of strengthening your abdominal and pelvic muscles for delivery and increasing your respiratory efficiency throughout your pregnancy.

## Chiropractic Medicine

Therapeutic manipulation of the skeleton, particularly of the spine, was commonly used by Greek physicians as early as the fourth century A.D. Chiropractic, meaning "done by hand" in Greek, was developed by Daniel David Palmer, who performed his first spinal adjustment in 1895 and claimed that he used it to cure a patient of deafness. Palmer deduced that the nervous system was the ultimate control mechanism of the body and that the adjustment of even minor misalignments of the spine (which he called *subluxations*) could safely and effectively relieve many disorders.

Chiropractic has been used to treat a variety of normal but, nevertheless, uncomfortable conditions during pregnancy, including fatigue, morning sickness, heartburn, headaches, neck pain, back pain, and labor pain.

## Homeopathy

Homeopathy was founded in the late eighteenth century by the German physician Samuel Hahnemann, who discovered that very small, diluted doses of certain botanical medicines can stimulate the body's immune system to combat illness. As a result, he prescribed remedies to enhance rather than suppress symptoms. Homeopathy is based on the *law of similars,* which states that any substance capable of making you ill may also cure you if it is administered in a dose that is small enough to treat the symptoms. The homeopathic remedies recommended for pregnancy, labor, and the postpartum period are widely considered safe and effective, but you should always discuss them with your caregiver or homeopath before using them.

A homeopathic remedy is prepared by repeatedly diluting a substance and shaking it vigorously between dilutions. The shaking process, known as succussion, releases the healing power of the substance; the dilution process minimizes its side effects. The more diluted the remedy, the more potent it becomes, so only a minute quantity is needed to be effective.

Homeopathic remedies have been used to treat a variety of problems during pregnancy, including nausea, vomiting, respiratory and digestive disorders, urinary problems, anemia, fluid retention, and slightly elevated blood pressure. Homeopathic remedies may also be beneficial during childbirth. A Swiss study conducted by Bernard Hochstrasser found that pregnant women with anemia experienced "fewer hemorrhages and decreased abnormal contractions" during labor when they were given homeopathic remedies instead of conventional drugs.

## Hydrotherapy

Hydrotherapy was developed in 1820 by Dr. Vincenz Priessnitz, who collected data on the healing powers of water and temperature change. Methods of hydrotherapy include sitz (sitting) baths, douches, spas and hot tubs, whirlpools, saunas, showers, immersion baths, poultices, and foot baths.

Hydrotherapy has been proven effective in relieving many discomforts associated with elevated blood pressure and pressure against the spine during the late stages of pregnancy. A study conducted by Dr. Dean Edell found that taking a bath in 92°F water fifty minutes a day for five days relieved edema, the normal but uncomfortable swelling that results from water retention during pregnancy. Be sure to consult with your caregiver before starting any water immersion program, and avoid immersing yourself in water (including baths) that is hotter than 96°F.

## Hypnosis

In their book, *Beyond Biofeedback,* Elmer and Alyce Green of the Menninger Clinic describe a patient with a painful pelvic tumor the size of a grapefruit. The patient was hypnotized and told to find the "room" in his brain that had the valves controlling the blood supply to his body and to mentally "turn off" the valve that controlled the blood flow to his tumor. He did so, and within two months of hypnosis therapy, the tumor shrank to one fourth its original size.

Several childbirth courses, including the ASPO/Lamaze and Bradley methods, incorporate hypnosis in their methods of preparing women for childbirth (see Chapter 5). Hypnosis can help you cope with pain and fear throughout pregnancy and childbirth. By helping you convert negative images into positive visualizations, it can also be used effectively to relieve stress or help you give up smoking or drinking alcohol. You will also find it helpful for relieving headaches, facial neuralgia, and sciatica. Hypnosis has even been used in place of local anesthesia during cesarean deliveries (see Chapter 11).

## Intimacy

Your feelings of intimacy with your partner can also affect your baby's development, because a fetus can sense your emotions. Arguments and conflicts or a lack of social support can stimulate the release of *stress hormones,* which are transferred through your blood to your fetus. Research has shown, for example, that infants born to mothers who are under emotional stress due to marital problems or the absence of the baby's father are more likely to develop colic than infants born to mothers with a supportive social environment.

An intimate relationship with your partner, on the other hand, will help you maintain the *relaxation response* and, thus, strengthen your immune system. Research studies show that people who feel loved and supported by their partners tend to develop healthier personal habits, such as relaxing more and maintaining a healthy diet. The results of such habits include fewer illnesses and infections.

Throughout this book, we stress the emotional as well as physical changes that you'll experience during pregnancy and childbirth. If you're single, it's extremely important that you enjoy the intimacy and support of your family and close friends throughout your pregnancy. Besides accompanying you to your monthly checkups and childbirth education classes, they can lend an ear when you need to talk about your concerns and fears. Someone close to you can also act as a coach, supporter, and advocate during labor and childbirth.

## Massage

Human touch has long been recognized as a powerful healing agent, soothing and even curing many physical discomforts of pregnancy. In India and Japan, massage is an important part of a midwife's training and is used to prepare both mother and baby for birth and the postnatal period.

A full body massage stimulates nerve endings in the skin and the amniotic sac and improves the flow of blood and lymph so that oxygen, nutrients, and waste products can be transported more efficiently. It will also help lower your heart rate and blood pressure.

Massage is especially effective in relieving pain during labor, because it stimulates the release of endorphins. The Bradley and ASPO/Lamaze childbirth programs teach pregnant women to massage the *perineum* (the small space between the anus and the vagina) before delivery to prevent pain and reduce the risk of tearing during delivery.

## Meditation

Dr. Bernie Siegel's book, *Love, Medicine & Miracles,* defines meditation as "an active process of focusing the mind into a state of relaxed awareness." In our book, you'll find a description of several different types of meditation, including methods that focus attention on sound (mantras), on images (mandalas), and on breathing.

The purpose of all meditation methods, according to Siegel, is ultimately the same: "to induce a restful trance which strengthens the mind by freeing it from its accustomed turmoil." He notes that meditation lowers or normalizes blood pressure, pulse rate, and stress hormone levels in the blood. It can also help lower abnormally high cholesterol levels, increase your ability to concentrate, heighten your sense of personal happiness, overcome negative thinking, and reduce anger.

## Nutrition and Supplements

Socrates once said, "There is only one good, knowledge, and one evil, ignorance." His observation is certainly true about nutrition during pregnancy, because the nutrients you do (or don't) consume help determine your health and the health of your baby. Your food intake during the first days of pregnancy is crucial, because the only way the child in your womb can receive the nutrients and oxygen it needs for growth is from your blood. If your diet lacks essential nutrients, it can cause irreversible damage that may not become fully apparent until your child is born or reaches maturity.

The safest way to ensure that you're getting the nutrients your child requires is to have your caregiver evaluate your food intake on a regular basis. In Chapter 3, we provide an outline of a nutritional program for each trimester based on the Recommended Dietary Allowances (RDAs) developed by the National Food and Nutrition Board.

Vitamins and minerals are essential chemical compounds; that is, they must be included in your diet to ensure the healthy growth of your baby. They are only needed in small amounts to build, maintain, and repair tissues, and are usually available in diets that feature a variety of fresh fruits and vegetables. In Chapter 3, we describe the essential vitamins and minerals you need during pregnancy, what each does for your body, and which foods contain them.

Along with diet, nutrition therapy (the use of vitamin and mineral supplements) is effective for relieving many of the discomforts and complications of pregnancy. We recommend taking supplements of essential nutrients, including vitamins C, B complex, and folic acid (vitamin $B_9$), and the minerals zinc, iron, calcium, and magnesium if you cannot consume adequate amounts of nutrient-rich foods. Our recommendations appear in Chapter 4.

## Osteopathic Medicine

Because several of his own children died from drug overdoses, Andrew Taylor Still, an American Civil War physician, developed a new therapy called *osteopathy* or bone treatment. Still believed that many diseases could be healed by manipulating bones and joints (especially in the cranium and spine) to increase blood circulation and improve nerve function. Still was able to find positions and movements to adjust (or *crack*) most of the larger joints of the body.

Osteopathy has been used to relieve spinal and joint pain, sciatica, allergies, breathing problems, fatigue, and headaches, and to lower blood pressure. Cranial osteopathy is considered especially helpful for relieving pain due to sore or tight pelvic, spinal, or neck muscles during pregnancy. It's also helpful for relieving depression, insomnia, and physical or psychological stress. Your newborn baby may also benefit from osteopathy if its skull or spine were traumatized during birth. Furthermore, since doctors of osteopathy (D.O.s) have medical degrees, they can help resolve other concerns that arise during pregnancy.

## Physical Activity

Giving birth to a baby is a high-endurance physical activity that will severely strain most of the skeletal muscles in your body. The better your physical condition throughout pregnancy, the less stressful your labor and childbirth will be. Studies have shown that women who exercise during pregnancy experience fewer complications and less pain during labor.

In Chapter 4, we provide guidelines for a safe and effective program of exercise throughout your pregnancy. Even if you did not exercise regularly before you became pregnant, you can safely begin this workout now. The most beneficial first-time physical activities for pregnant women include swimming, yoga, and brisk walking, because they are safe and help maintain circulation, strengthen your abdominal muscles, and may relieve many discomforts of pregnancy, including cramps, fatigue, headaches, varicose veins, and a variety of muscle aches and pains.

## Qigong

For muscular and cardiovascular conditioning, poise, balance, breathing, relaxation—and yes, even the ability to bust a board with your bare hands—martial arts, such as qigong, offer incredible benefits. They help you channel energy throughout your body to help you relax and breathe more efficiently. Many studies have proven that qigong reduces heart rate, blood pressure, depressive episodes, and addiction, and triggers the release of endorphins.

Qigong (pronounced *chee gong*) is an ancient Chinese exercise that combines calisthenics movements with breathing to stimulate the flow of qi (pronounced *chi*), the vital life energy that flows through the acupuncture meridians (energy pathways). Several variations of qigong are helpful during pregnancy and labor. In the first form, you sit in a relaxed pose and use your mental energy to channel your qi to specific parts of your body, especially your womb. In the second form, breathing meditations are coordinated with graceful, dance-like movements that also channel qi through the meridians. Today, most hospitals in China include qigong as part of their prenatal programs.

## Traditional Chinese Medicine (TCM)

According to an old Chinese prayer, "When you have a disease, do not try to cure it. Find your chi and you will be healed." In traditional Chinese medicine (TCM), foods, herbs, acupuncture, acupressure, tai chi, moxibustion (application of heat to acupuncture points), and massage are used to increase or decrease the flow of chi as needed.

Traditional Chinese medicine is also useful if you develop cramps during pregnancy caused by chi stagnation (the inability of vital energy to move freely through the body) in the lower abdomen, blood stasis (blood pooling), or a combination of both. It has also been used to relieve insomnia and shrink varicose veins.

## Visualization Methods

Siegel's *Love, Medicine & Miracles* reported a clinical trial in which a young boy with an inoperable brain tumor used visualization to make his tumor disappear. He learned self-regulation techniques that helped him "control his body with his mind, imagining for example, rockets ships flying around in his head shooting at the tumor." This simple form of imagery induced his immune system to attack and eventually eliminate his tumor.

If we can vividly imagine we're relaxing, we—like Siegel's patient —can guide our brain into doing it, thus inducing the relaxation response. Several visualization exercises that are important during pregnancy and childbirth are described in this book. Studies have shown that mothers who have negative and fearful images of labor and childbirth tend to have upset, colicky babies. Mothers who visualize positive images before birth tend to have calmer babies and enjoy more satisfying relationships with their children after birth.

## Yoga

Pregnancy is an incredible miracle—a very *physical* miracle. Virtually every part of your body will undergo physiological changes. Hormonal secretions will relax and soften the ligaments that hold your joints together to allow them to expand in preparation for birth. Your body fluid levels will increase by 20 percent, and your heart will work harder to ensure that the increased blood volume is pumped throughout your body so that an adequate supply reaches the placenta as well as your own vital organs. The workload for your kidneys also increases because the kidneys filter blood and excrete waste products for both you and your baby. In addition, your digestion slows down as hormones soften the muscles of the digestive tract.

The yoga exercises outlined in this book will help increase your rates of circulation, elimination, and respiration and improve your energy level. The meaning of the word yoga is *union*—the integration of physical, mental, and spiritual energies. Yoga involves many different forms of physical (stretching), breathing, and mental exercises. Some yoga practices also incorporate visualization, progressive relaxation exercises, and meditation. In Chapter 5, we describe several yoga exercises that gently relieve back, neck, and joint pain, and automatically regulate your heartbeat and breathing.

As you gradually discover a greater degree of suppleness and freedom of movement, you will become increasingly comfortable in positions and movements that are natural to labor and gain confidence in your ability to cope with painful contractions. When the time comes to give birth, you will know instinctively how to use your body, letting it flow with the contractions and enabling your pelvis to expand more easily as your baby moves through the birth canal.

## GETTING STARTED

The Chinese have an ancient saying about the wisdom of "walking on both feet," which means using the best of Eastern and Western medical procedures. "Walking on both feet" aptly describes the holistic approach to pregnancy and childbirth presented in this book. The suggestions presented here form a comprehensive, safe, and clinically proven program. Your miraculous journey toward childbirth is about to begin.

## Chapter 2

# The First Month

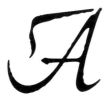

MIRACLE HAS OCCURRED!

A brand new baby is on its way. Your partner's sperm has fertilized one of your eggs (called an *ovum*) as it traveled down one of your fallopian tubes, thus creating a new human being. The fertilized egg began to divide into the many cells that will form your baby's organs, even before it became implanted in the lining of your uterus. By the end of the first month, the *embryo* will already be three centimeters long and have the faint outline of a human body. It will also develop a rudimentary nervous system and a primitive heart which will begin to pulsate and circulate blood.

Now that you know you're pregnant, you probably have lots of questions and concerns, which we will try to answer in this chapter. Your most important considerations this month should be deciding where you want to have your baby, developing your Birth Plan, and choosing your caregiver. Sounds like a lot to think about, but this chapter will help guide you through it. We'll give you advice on how to preview birth sites, draw up a Birth Plan Worksheet, and interview and choose your caregiver. We will also provide a checkup form for you to take to your first monthly visit with your selected caregiver.

You should note that this book divides pregnancy into months rather than weeks (as doctors do) because most women keep track of their pregnancies this way. Keep in mind that the first month of your pregnancy is considered the first thirty days beginning seven days after the first day of your last menstrual period. If, for example, your last menstrual period began on January 1, your first month began on January 8. Your second month would then begin on February 8, your third on March 8, and so on. You can calculate your estimated delivery date by adding nine months and seven days to the first day of your last normal menstrual period. So your estimated due date (EDD) would be nine months later, on September 8.

# ESPECIALLY *for* FATHERS

CONGRATULATIONS! YOU'RE GOING TO BE A FATHER. You've probably already found that pregnancy is a time of change—for your partner, for you, and for your relationship. Understanding these changes and knowing how to cope with them will help you enjoy this special time in your life.

Your role as a father can begin long before your baby is born. Research suggests that women with supportive partners have fewer health problems during pregnancy and more positive feelings about their changing bodies. Studies also show that labor and delivery are easier and shorter for women whose partners take part in the process. So now is the time to get involved.

One way to get involved is by attending your partner's monthly checkups. At each visit, your partner will be weighed and tests will be performed to monitor the progress of the pregnancy. Her caregiver will check fetal activity and assess the growth and health of your baby by measuring the woman's abdomen and listening to the fetal heartbeat. Your caregiver will also tell you how best to promote a healthy holistic pregnancy and answer any questions you may have about your baby's growth, your partner's health, the birth process, and hospital procedures. Helping your partner fill in her monthly checkup form is a good way to support her and keep yourself informed about the miracle of childbirth!

# CHOOSING YOUR HOLISTIC CAREGIVER

Who you choose as a caregiver is perhaps *the* most important decision you will make during your pregnancy. Remember, your caregiver is an intimate partner in your pregnancy, with equal responsibility for your health and the health of your baby. You want to be sure to choose someone who is not only qualified, competent, and who whole-heartedly believes in the holistic program for pregnancy and childbirth that you've chosen, but who you also trust completely and feel comfortable with. You have basically three options, which are reviewed below: an obstetrician, a family practitioner (FP), or a midwife.

## Obstetrician

If you have an underlying illness, such as diabetes, heart disease, or high blood pressure, or if you know you're a high-risk patient (as defined later in this chapter), then your caregiver should be an obstetrician who is trained to handle complications and emergencies during pregnancy, labor, and delivery. An obstetrician is a medical doctor who has had specialized training in pregnancy and childbirth. To become a specialist in obstetrics in the United States, a physician must pass a board certification examination administered by the American College of Obstetricians and Gynecologists (ACOG); in Canada, the examination is administered by the Royal College of Physicians and Surgeons. Obstetrician-gynecologists provide most of the maternity care in the United States.

The main disadvantage of using obstetricians is that they tend to recommend cesarean delivery, drugs during labor, and episiotomy more often than midwives or doulas.

Solo obstetricians work for themselves and usually use another doctor to care for their patients when they are unavailable. In partnerships or group practices, one or more doctors in the same specialty may see you for your monthly checkups on a rotating basis. The advantage of choosing a solo or group practice is that you will probably know the doctor who will deliver your baby. The disadvantage of partnerships and group practices is that you may not like all the doctors, and you won't be able to choose the one who attends your delivery. You may also receive conflicting advice from various partners.

Another alternative is a practice that includes one or more obstetricians and nurse-midwives. With this option, you also have the disadvantage of not necessarily knowing who will attend your delivery. You will have the advantage of having, in effect, two caregivers: a licensed nurse-midwife, trained in obstetrics and familiar with the holistic practices used by midwives, who can be your labor and delivery coach; and an obstetrician with hospital privileges, who is trained for emergencies if complications arise. In many ways, this is an ideal situation.

## Family Practitioner

The family practitioner is similar to the traditional general practitioner (GP)—except the family practitioner has had several years of specialty training in primary care, including obstetrics, after receiving an M.D. Family physicians are thus trained to care for pregnant women, as well as other family members, from infancy through old age, although they usually refer high-risk maternity cases to obstetricians or perinatologists. Family physicians provide most of the maternity care in Canada.

The advantage to choosing a family practitioner is that he or she can serve both as your caregiver during pregnancy and your pediatrician after delivery. In addition, you may already know the caregiver personally if he or she has attended other members of your family. Ideally, the family practitioner will be interested in all aspects of your health, not just your pregnancy, and will view pregnancy as just a normal part of the life cycle rather than as an illness. The disadvantage is that if complications occur, your family practitioner may have to call in a specialist for consultation or perhaps to deliver your baby, and you will probably not know that individual.

## Certified Nurse-Midwife

If your pregnancy is low-risk and you already know that you want a natural birth in a birthing center or even at home, you'll probably want to select a certified nurse-midwife (CNM) as your caregiver.

In the United States, there are several categories of midwives: certified nurse-midwives, certified midwives (CMs), and lay midwives. A certified nurse-midwife is a registered nurse (RN) who has graduated from a midwifery program certified by the American College of Nurse Midwives. Many obtain a master's degree after completing their nurse-midwifery training. They usually practice with an obstetrician, although in some states they can deliver babies on their own. They usually have hospital privileges, but may also deliver babies in birthing centers or home settings. Care by a certified nurse-midwife is covered by most health plans and insurance programs.

The advantages of selecting a certified nurse-midwife is that she is a licensed nurse, experienced in obstetrics, trained in midwifery, and knowledgeable about holistic self-care—all of which means that she is more likely to treat your pregnancy as a natural process rather than as a medical emergency.

The November/December 1993 issue of *Natural Health* reports that a five-year study sponsored by the National Institutes of Health showed that women attended by certified nurse-midwives were less likely to have cesarean deliveries or episiotomies, or to be given sedatives or anesthesia. The researchers examined the birth records of children born to 800 women who delivered at the University of Michigan Hospital during a five-year period, some using certified nurse-midwives and others using physicians. Thirteen percent of midwife patients were given epidural anesthesia during labor compared with 41 percent of physician patients, 32 percent of midwife patients received episiotomies compared with 59 percent of physician patients, and only 8 percent of midwife patients required cesarean deliveries compared with 19 percent of physician patients.

Some American states and Canadian provinces allow certified midwives to deliver babies. Certified midwives receive training comparable with that provided by midwifery training programs in Europe, but they do not have a nursing degree. Instead, they usually take college courses and then complete a two- to three-year program in midwifery. Most licensed midwives practice outside the hospital, providing care for home births and birth-center births. Their orientation toward pregnancy and delivery, like that of certified nurse-midwives, is more holistic than that of the obstetrician or family practitioner.

Certified midwives usually practice in a hospital birth center or free-standing birth center and usually provide care for low-risk women, only. The disadvantage of choosing a certified midwife is that if complications arise during your pregnancy (they occur in approximately 20 percent of pregnancies), you may have to switch to an obstetrician and develop a patient–caregiver relationship all over again. Also, if an emergency arises during labor or delivery (which occurs 10 percent to 15 percent of the time), you may need the services of the obstetrician on call, who may be a stranger and may not want to use holistic alternatives. If complications arise at a free-standing maternity center, you may have to be transported to the nearest hospital for emergency care.

In some states, certified nurse-midwives and certified midwives may be unavailable, especially in rural areas, and a lay midwife may be your only alternative. *Lay midwives* usually receive informal training as apprentices to experienced midwives or participate in short courses, study groups, or independent study programs. Their qualifications, experiences, and standards of care vary. The primary advantage of using a lay midwife is that they tend to use holistic methods and are very sensitive to a prospective mother's wishes. Many are mothers themselves and are passionate about natural birth, so they will encourage you to have a home birth. They usually have excellent equipment and professional backup; however, they cannot attend high-risk pregnancies and will have to transfer you to an obstetrician in a hospital if complications develop during labor.

## Doulas

You might also consider hiring a doula, or birth attendant, as your secondary caregiver. *Doula* is Greek for "woman caregiver." Doulas provide many of the services of a midwife, including massage, encouragement, reassurance, and pain relief. If your partner takes an active role in your pregnancy and labor, he and your doula will work together.

A doula cannot be your primary caregiver, however, and she is not trained or licensed to attend high-risk women. Several studies have shown, however, that doulas provide excellent secondary assistance. Six different studies found that when a doula was present, labor was 25 percent shorter, requests for epidurals decreased by 60 percent, and women were half as likely to undergo cesarean deliveries. Some HMOs and health providers now cover the cost of a doula.

## CHOOSING YOUR HOLISTIC BIRTH SETTING

Ideally, while you're considering the type of caregiver you want, you should also be considering the type of birth setting (hospital, freestanding birth center, home birth, etc.) you want, as this will help you choose a caregiver who meets your requirements in that setting. Obviously, where you choose to have your baby will determine the alternatives that will be available to you during childbirth. The most important factor is to select one that provides an environment in which you feel safe, comfortable, and fully in control.

When it comes to birth settings, you have four basic options: a traditional hospital, a hospital birth center, a free-standing birth center (FSBC), or a home birth. You also have the option of a *water birth* (see below), which may be carried out in any of these settings. We suggest that you familiarize yourself with each option before choosing your caregiver. Read books, review videos, talk to friends, and, if possible, watch a real birth in each setting. The more you know about each option, the better.

At the moment, you may feel overwhelmed by the many decisions you have to make. If you like, skip ahead and read the birth scenarios at the end of this chapter. That'll give you a head start!

## Traditional Hospital Birth

If you live in a remote rural area and don't have access to a midwife, your only option may be a traditional hospital birth. In traditional hospitals, labor, delivery, and recovery usually take place in different rooms. The advantage of a traditional hospital birth, of course, is that if problems develop during labor or delivery, medical specialists are close at hand and sophisticated equipment is usually in the same room or just down the hall.

Studies show that the disadvantage of the traditional setting is that mothers have the *least* control over how they give birth in this setting. In a hospital, you're most likely to be confined to your bed during labor, to have intravenous (IV) lines and electronic monitors attached to you, to be given anesthetics for labor pain, and to be advised to have a cesarean delivery if minor complications develop.

Some hospitals have birthing suites as well as labor and delivery (LD) rooms and assign patients to whichever is available when they are admitted. Their policies vary on whether family members can remain with you throughout labor and delivery.

If this setting is realistically your only option, you'll need to be firm with the hospital about following your Birth Plan. We suggest that you give your caregiver a copy ahead of time and have your partner or advocate bring a copy when you are taken to the hospital. If you insist that the Plan is followed, you may be able to arrange an unrushed, family-oriented, noninterventional labor and delivery.

If you have more than one traditional hospital to choose from, you should visit all of them and ask for information on their rates for cesarean deliveries, drug administration, and episiotomies. You should also discuss your Birth Plan with them. This will give you a better idea of which hospital has the best environment for a holistic birth.

## Hospital Birthing Centers

Many hospitals now have family-centered birth centers with dual-purpose obstetrical suites called LDRs (Labor, Delivery, and Recovery), where women go through labor, delivery, and recovery. This makes it possible for a woman to stay in the same room, sometimes for the entire hospital stay, and for their babies to remain by their sides. The rooms are fully equipped for uncomplicated deliveries and for complications requiring noninvasive or minimally invasive procedures (in most hospitals, cesareans and other procedures are handled in a delivery or operating room). With all these precautions, they still look much like cozy bedrooms, with soft lighting and a comfortable bed that is usually used as the birthing bed. Most hospital birthing centers allow the father to be present during the birth.

The advantage of hospital birthing centers is that they are more holistic—they have lower cesarean, drug use, and episiotomy rates, and they encourage mothers to be the primary decision maker. Many centers work with you during your pregnancy to make sure you stay fit and follow a nutritious food plan. Some also offer childbirth classes and provide instruction on breastfeeding and basic infant care. In the most progressive centers, you are expected to take responsibility for your own health—weighing yourself, testing your own urine, even reviewing your own chart and recording the results of your monthly checkups.

One disadvantage of hospital birthing centers is that state licensing laws prevent them from admitting high-risk women. Also, the rates for cesareans, drug administration, and episiotomies are higher than they are at free-standing births centers (FSBCs) or during home births.

## Free-Standing Birth Centers

A variation of hospital family-centered care is the *free-standing birth center* (FSBC), which is affiliated with but may not be governed by a major hospital. Most of these facilities use a comanagement model of care wherein a midwife provides most of the care during pregnancy and childbirth, but an obstetrician is called in if the midwife encounters any problems. In a study by James Rooks that was published in the August 1989 issue of the *New England Journal of Medicine,* women who gave birth in free-standing birth centers needed less anesthesia, had fewer episiotomies and cesarean deliveries, and went home earlier than women who delivered in a hospital. The average stay in a free-standing birth center after delivery is seven hours.

Because they are usually close to emergency care, some free-standing birth centers accept patients with minor complications. Women seeking a vaginal birth after a previous cesarean delivery and those with diet-controlled gestational diabetes (diabetes that develops during pregnancy), for example, may be acceptable candidates.

Free-standing birth centers offer a compromise between hospital births and home births. They provide a homelike setting—so your friends and relatives can be present during the birth, if you choose—and they have some emergency equipment in case you have complications. They each have different policies regarding the circumstances under which they will transfer a mother to a hospital, so be sure to ask about them during your visit. According to Rooks, only 15 to 20 percent of first-time mothers who choose a free-standing birth center need to be transferred to a hospital during labor or after delivery.

Another advantage of the free-standing birth center is that they let you have two caregivers: an obstetrician, who will be on call when you go into labor; and a certified nurse-midwife, who will examine you each month and act as your labor coach. If both are trained in holistic medicine, you'll be in good hands.

## Home Births

Women have been having babies at home for centuries. Studies show that home births are perfectly safe for low-risk women as long as they're attended by a trained caregiver—usually a midwife or nurse, or occasionally an obstetrician. Proponents claim that home births are as safe, if not safer, than hospital births in terms of the risk for birth injuries, maternal hemorrhaging, and the need for intervention.

Each caregiver will have his or her own criteria for evaluating each patient for a home delivery. Many obstetricians and certified nurse-midwives will not perform a home delivery for twins, a breech baby, or a first-time mother over the age of thirty-five. Be sure to ask your caregiver during your initial interview about the criteria he or she uses. If you're considering a certified nurse-midwife or certified midwife as the primary caregiver at your home birth, make sure she has a state license to do so. Some certified nurse-midwives and obstetricians may choose not to attend home births because of malpractice insurance or a lack of emergency backup.

The problem with having a home birth is that if something goes wrong, the facilities for an emergency cesarean delivery or resuscitation of the newborn may not be close at hand. If you want a home birth, you should have a low-risk pregnancy and you should choose a well-trained caregiver who's experienced with emergencies and has hospital privileges. Also, your home should be reasonably close to a fully equipped, modern hospital.

## Water Births

Water births were pioneered in France by Dr. Michel Odent and have become increasingly popular in the United States. Mothers go through labor and deliver their baby in a sanitized tub. Advocates claim that this is the easiest way to give birth, for both mother and baby, because it shortens labor and makes pushing easier. They also claim that birthing in water reduces the risk of perineal tearing.

Most obstetricians and hospital administrators, however, feel that the risks of water birth outweigh its benefits. As a result, many hospitals do not offer it as an alternative. Some caregivers, including midwives, will not perform water births because of the risks to the baby, which include the possibility that the baby will not breathe quickly enough on its own or will become infected by the contaminants in the tub water. Both risks can be controlled, however. If you want a water birth, find a free-standing birth center that offers it. If you want one at home, you'll have to find a caregiver who is licensed to offer it.

# Your Holistic Birth Plan

By now you should have chosen your birth site and have some idea of the type of holistic caregiver you prefer. Now's the time to finalize your Birth Plan, which is basically a written description of your priorities and preferred options during labor, birth, and afterward. When you build a new house, you work from a set of blueprints. The blueprints are often revised, but nevertheless indicate what each contractor is supposed to do. Similarly, a Birth Plan is a written statement of how you would like to deliver your baby. It may be placed in your medical chart where it can be read and consulted by everyone involved in your care.

The more detailed your Birth Plan, the better. You'll find that some caregivers will be more enthusiastic about your Birth Plan than others. You'll need a caregiver who will follow it as much as possible and consult you before making any changes to it. We have included below a Birth Plan Worksheet that lists important concerns that you should discuss with your caregiver and the birth site administrator. Filling out the worksheet will ensure that you and your caregivers are on the same page from the beginning of your pregnancy. If you prefer, skip ahead to the chapters on labor, delivery, and postpartum care to familiarize yourself with standard procedures in different birth sites.

Keep in mind that hospital rules and your caregiver's advice may cause you to change your Plan. Since there's no way to predict precisely how labor and delivery will progress, your original Birth Plan may not always be in the best interest of you or your baby, and last-minute changes may be necessary. If so, try to be flexible and keep in mind that the priorities in any birth should always be the health and safety of the mother and child.

## Interviewing Your Caregiver

Once you've filled out your worksheet, you're ready to interview potential caregivers. We suggest that you begin by shopping over the phone. You can ask the telephone receptionist basic questions about the candidate's background, for example, his or her education, training, number of years in practice, number of births attended, and hospital privileges. You can also find out the cost of care, the insurance plans that are accepted, and holistic therapies that are practiced. Be sure to ask the candidates how much time they allow for each monthly appointment and who will see you if your primary caregiver is not available.

Once you've screened potential caregivers by phone, you can make appointments to interview those who are likely to meet your basic requirements in person. During each interview, you should discuss each item on your Birth Plan worksheet and find out how the caregiver feels about anything that is of particular concern to you. That way you won't have any unpleasant last-minute surprises.

# $\mathcal{H}$OLISTIC BIRTH PLAN WORKSHEET

Questions to ask your birth site administrator and caregiver:

***Labor***  Can I have a home birth? _____

How far into labor can I remain at home? _____

Can I walk about or sit up during labor?_____

Can I bring a squatting stool? _____

Can I wear my own clothes?_____

Can I have music, flowers, and personal items from home in my room? _____

Can I photograph or videotape the delivery? _____

Can my partner stay with me during labor and delivery? _____

Which holistic methods do you use for labor?

    Hypnosis_____

    Transcutaneous Electrical Nerve Stimulation (TENS)_____

    Acupuncture _____

    Physical Therapy_____

    Other_____

Under what circumstances do you recommend:

    enemas during labor?_____

    intravenous fluids? _____

    catheterization? _____

    pain medication?_____

    artificial rupture of membranes? _____

    drugs to stimulate labor? _____

    shaving of pubic area? _____

    analgesics? _____

    general anesthesia?_____

    tranquilizers? _____

    inhalants?_____

    caudal block?_____

    saddle block? _____

    epidurals?_____

Is a full-time anesthetist available who is qualified to administer epidurals?_____

| | |
|---|---|
| *Delivery* | Can I choose my delivery position(s)? _____ |
| | Under what circumstances do you recommend: |
| | episiotomies?_____ |
| | vacuum extraction? _____ |
| | cesarean delivery? _____ |
| | Can my partner cut the umbilical cord?_____ |
| | |
| *Postpartum* | Can I breastfeed immediately following delivery? _____ |
| | Can silver nitrate eye drops or erythromycin ointment application be postponed until after I have bonded with my baby?_____ |
| | Are any postpartum medication or treatments required? _____ |
| | How soon after giving birth can I leave the hospital if there are no complications? _____ |
| | Who will determine my baby's feeding schedule while we are in the hospital? _____ |
| | If I have to stay in the hospital for more than a day after delivery, can my partner stay with me? _____ |

You should ask the potential caregiver about the diagnostic procedures and interventions they normally use during labor. Do all patients receive intravenous fluids and electronic fetal monitoring? Are women free to walk, move freely, and take showers during labor? What about the use of medication and anesthesia? Under what circumstances does the caregiver perform a cesarean delivery or episiotomy? When and how is labor induced? Does the caregiver recommend enemas? Under what circumstances is a forceps delivery performed?

Other questions might center on the caregiver's attitude towards the father's or partner's participation in a normal labor and delivery or a cesarean birth. Are other support people also welcome? When does the caregiver usually arrive during labor? How much time does he or she spend with the patient during labor? Who provides professional support and care during labor in your caregiver's absence?

If you're planning a home birth, you will want to know what equipment will be brought for normal care and for emergencies and what the caregiver's criteria are for transferring you to a hospital if problems arise. Can the caregiver continue to provide your care in the hospital? Will the caregiver (if not an obstetrician) remain as a support person and advocate if a hospital obstetrician takes over the management of your case? Will your caregiver accompany you to the hospital in case of complications or an emergency?

## THE FIRST-MONTH CHECKUP

Ideally, you will have discussed your Birth Plan with your caregiver before your first-month checkup. During the checkup, your caregiver will confirm your pregnancy, record your medical history, and examine your cervix and uterus to determine the approximate age of your pregnancy and look for any gross abnormalities. If you haven't already had one, a pregnancy test may be ordered.

Bring all your home records to the checkup, including items pertaining to your personal medical history (a list of chronic illnesses, previous major illnesses, or surgery; medications you're currently taking or have taken since conception; any known allergies, including drug allergies; your family medical history (genetic disorders, such as Tay-Sachs disease, sickle cell anemia, thalassemia, or Down syndrome; and chronic diseases such as hypertension, diabetes, heart disease, or respiratory problems); personal habits, such as smoking, drinking, exercise, and diet; your gynecologic and obstetrical history (age at which first menstruation began; duration and regularity of menstrual periods; abortions, miscarriages, stillbirths, and live births; and any problems during past pregnancies); and factors in your personal life, such as work or an impending separation or divorce, that you think might affect your pregnancy.

## FILLING OUT YOUR MONTHLY CHECKUP FORM

We strongly recommend that you keep your own record of each monthly checkup. This type of diary will help increase your knowledge of what's happening to your body. The more information you

## THE PHYSICAL EXAMINATION

Your physical examination is designed to evaluate any or all of the following:

▷ Heart and lungs

▷ Breasts and abdomen

▷ Blood pressure, to serve as a baseline for comparison at subsequent visits

▷ Height and weight, also to serve as a baseline

▷ Extremities, for signs of varicose veins and edema (swelling due to fluid buildup)

▷ External genitalia (labia majora and minora)

▷ Vagina and cervix, using a speculum

▷ Pelvic organs, by means of a bimanual exam (with one hand in the vagina and one on the abdomen) and also by finger palpation (touch) through the rectum and vagina

▷ Bony pelvis, for size and shape

Here's what your caregiver will be looking for:

▷ **Birth canal.** In some women, the passageway from the uterus through the vagina to the outside is too small for a normal vaginal birth, and a cesarean delivery may be required. Recognizing this problem early in pregnancy will allow your caregiver to plan for the procedure.

▷ **Blood Pressure.** High blood pressure (hypertension) can exist prior to pregnancy or develop as a complication of pregnancy. If left untreated, it can progress to *eclampsia*, a condition that can result in coma or death; therefore, high blood pressure should be diagnosed and treated as early as possible.

▷ **Weight.** Adequate weight gain is crucial for a successful pregnancy. Ask your caregiver to recommend a food plan that is appropriate for your ideal body weight early in pregnancy.

▷ **Fundus Examination.** Your abdomen should be examined each month to determine the location of the top of the uterus (fundus), which is where implantation usually occurs. Uterine growth that's too rapid or too slow may indicate abnormal fetal development and should be investigated further.

▷ **Fetal Heart Rate.** Your baby's heart rate should also be monitored each month to ensure that it is in a normal range (about 120 to 150 beats per minute). If more than one heart rate is heard, it implies multiple birth (such as twins or triplets).

record, the more you'll know; and the more you know, the more in control you'll feel. Studies have shown that mothers who feel more in control of their pregnancy have more positive memories of labor and delivery and report less pain and depression after delivery. We've included Monthly Checkup forms in Appendix A.

# COMMON PRENATAL TESTS

Under normal circumstances, extensive internal examinations are not necessary during your first monthly checkup, although your caregiver may order them toward the end of your pregnancy to re-evaluate your pelvic measurements, the position of your baby, the status of your cervix, and your expected delivery date. Some tests are routine for every pregnant woman; some are given more routinely in some areas of the country by certain practitioners, and some are performed only when warranted by special circumstances. The following are the most common prenatal tests:

▷ **Urinalysis.** This test looks for the amount of sugar, protein, white blood cells, and bacteria in the urine. *Sugar* (glucose) in the urine may indicate diabetes, which may have existed before pregnancy or may develop as a complication of pregnancy (gestational diabetes). *Protein* in the urine may be a sign of hypertension or kidney disease, both of which may complicate the pregnancy. Bacteria or white blood cells indicate infection such as a urinary tract infection, which frequently occurs during pregnancy.

▷ **Hematocrit.** *Hematocrit* is the concentration of red blood cells in the blood. A low hematocrit indicates anemia—often iron-deficiency anemia—which causes fatigue and makes it difficult to fight infections. It can also compromise the growth of your baby. Many women become anemic during pregnancy, and the hematocrit will detect this problem quickly so that appropriate treatment can be initiated.

▷ **Blood Glucose.** Because diabetes is common and may develop during pregnancy, most doctors screen routinely for glucose ("blood sugar") using a glucose tolerance test. Some caregivers administer the test monthly; others only use it once.

▷ **Tests for Sexually Transmitted Diseases.** While you're pregnant, you're at a slightly greater risk of contracting sexually transmitted viruses, such as cytomegalovirus, herpes virus, and AIDS, and it's extremely important that you and your sexual partner be tested to make sure you're not carrying any of them. Several sexually transmitted diseases, including syphilis and gonorrhea, can cause serious birth defects. Some of them can be treated without endangering your pregnancy if they are detected early enough.

▷ **Rubella Antibody Titer.** This tests for rubella (German measles), which can cause fatal birth defects, especially during the first trimester.

▷ **Pap Smear.** In addition to checking for cervical cancer, this test can also reveal the presence of an active genital herpes infection, which can cause serious problems— including the death of the baby if you have a vaginal delivery when the herpes is in an active phase. If the risk is great, your caregiver may advise you to have a cesarean delivery.

▷ **Vaginal–Cervix Culture.** Infection with bacteria called Group B *Streptococcus* (a cousin of the bacteria that cause strep throat) can cause pneumonia, meningitis, and death of the newborn if it is transmitted from mother to baby during delivery. It can easily be treated with penicillin or other antibiotics.

▷ **Genetic Screening.** This is an optional test for women or their partners who have a genetic predisposition for certain diseases, such as thalassemia, Tay-Sachs disease, sickle cell anemia, or Down syndrome.

— **Sickle cell anemia.** Sickle cell anemia is caused by an abnormal hemoglobin (the oxygen-carrying component of blood) that causes blood cells to change shape and results in a severe anemia and related complications. African-American women should have this test performed, because approximately 10 percent of African Americans carry the gene for this disease.

— **Tay-Sachs disease.** This disease is caused by an enzyme deficiency that results in the buildup of toxic materials in the nervous tissue, which can be fatal. The gene is carried by approximately 5 percent of Ashkenazi Jews.

— **Thalassemia.** This disease is caused by the genetic inability to make a key component of hemoglobin, and results in a form of anemia that can be fatal. This disorder is most common in people of Mediterranean descent as well as Asians, especially Chinese. Approximately 10 to 25 percent of people in these high-risk groups carry the gene for thalassemia.

## COMMON FIRST-MONTH CONCERNS

**High-Risk Pregnancies**

If your pregnancy is considered low risk, you are probably going to deliver a healthy baby. However, even low-risk pregnancies can develop problems later that move them into a high-risk category. For example, some healthy women develop diabetes or hypertension during their pregnancy, others develop an unusual pattern of weight gain (too rapid, too slow, or marked by sudden fluctuations), others do not deliver by two weeks after the due date, and still others experience abnormal uterine or vaginal bleeding. Fortunately, with the use of medical technology, pregnant women can be monitored carefully for signs and symptoms of high-risk conditions.

*Complications* are medical conditions, such as diabetes, that arise during pregnancy, labor, delivery, or after delivery which may place the mother or baby at risk. They may or may not resolve with treatment. Left untreated, however, they usually lead to an emergency.

*Emergencies* are situations that place the mother or baby in immediate danger and require immediate treatment to prevent the death of the mother or baby. For example, pregnancy-induced hypertension (PIH) is a complication which, if left untreated, can result in eclampsia in the mother, which can lead to coma or death.

## Miscarriage

Every expectant mother worries about miscarriage—usually unnecessarily, because fewer than 10 percent of all pregnant women miscarry after pregnancy has been diagnosed. Another 20 to 40 percent

---

### HIGH-RISK PREGNANCIES

Different caregivers define *high-risk pregnancies* differently. Any of the following factors may cause complications during your pregnancy. You should discuss them with your caregiver during your first-month checkup:

1. A medical history of heart disease, high blood pressure, diabetes, anemia, cancer, abnormal thyroid activity, multiple sclerosis, drug abuse, or alcoholism

2. Being more than thirty-five years of age or less than sixteen years of age

3. Being very overweight or underweight for your height

4. Previous history of cesarean delivery, forceps delivery, miscarriage, abortion, stillbirth, premature birth, prolonged labor, uterine bleeding during pregnancy, multiple births, or difficulty in conceiving

5. In this pregnancy, having high blood pressure, multiple fetuses, uterine bleeding, viral infection, abnormal fetal heart rate, unusual weight gain or weight loss, or gestational diabetes (diabetes developing during pregnancy)

6. Malnutrition

7. Organ damage, including liver problems such as cirrhosis and hepatitis; intestinal surgery, Crohn's disease (ulcerative colitis); chronic kidney infection (pyelitis or nephritis) or damage (nephrosis); kidney transplants or dialysis; heart disease; glandular disorders (including abnormal thyroid, pituitary, or adrenal gland activity); or asthma, emphysema, and other pulmonary disorders

8. Sexually transmitted diseases, including AIDS

9. Potentially disabling disorders, such as epilepsy, multiple sclerosis, or cerebral palsy

10. Cancer

of pregnancies end before a pregnancy diagnosis is made; these are the miscarriages that usually go unnoticed.

According to Gillespie in *Your Pregnancy: Month by Month,* national studies show that more than 95 percent of miscarriages are caused by genetic defects. The most common time for miscarriages, Gillespie states, is the eleventh to twelfth week. The next most likely time is the seventh week. Less than 3 percent of women who reach the sixteenth week of pregnancy miscarry before the twenty-eighth week.

## F A C T S    A B O U T    M I S C A R R I A G E

### Factors That Increase the Risk of Miscarriage

1. Genetic errors

2. Implantation errors due to genetic factors or a malformed uterus

3. Exposure of the fetus to radiation or harmful drugs

4. High fever

5. An intrauterine device (IUD) in place during conception

6. Scars on the cervix due to multiple abortions or other scarring procedures

7. Chronic maternal illness

8. Exposure of mother to rubella (German measles)

### Factors That Do Not Cause Miscarriages

1. IUD-related complications. Scarring of the endometrium (the lining of the uterus) by an IUD-triggered infection can prevent implantation, but usually does not cause miscarriage once implantation is established.

2. History of multiple abortions that has not resulted in cervical scarring. Multiple abortions can cause scarring of the endometrium which, like an IUD, can cause an endometrial infection but not necessarily a miscarriage.

3. Emotional distress resulting from an argument, family problems, or stress at work.

4. A minor fall or accident. Serious injuries, such as those sustained in an automobile accident or a serious fall (especially when the mother becomes unconscious), can, however, cause a miscarriage.

5. Normal physical activity, such as housework; lifting groceries, children, or other heavy objects; hanging curtains; moving light furniture; and moderate, safe exercise.

6. Sexual intercourse, unless the woman has a history of miscarriage or is otherwise at high risk for pregnancy loss.

*Symptoms of Miscarriage*

Most miscarriages begin with cramping in the lower abdomen and/or bleeding from the uterus. Miscarriage is inevitable if it is accompanied by both bleeding and dilation (widening) of the cervix. In some cases, bleeding begins with spotting; in others, it starts with severe hemorrhaging. Spotting and cramping before the twenty-fifth week are signs of a *threatened abortion.* If ultrasound shows a viable pregnancy, the mother may be advised to stay in bed for a few days. The cramping often halts and the pregnancy usually proceeds normally. If you experience cramps or bleeding, call your caregiver immediately.

*Preventing Miscarriages*

Our Holistic Program for Pregnancy and Childbirth stresses prevention of complications and emergencies through sound nutrition, regular exercise, and relaxation. The more closely you follow the

---

## POSSIBLE SIGNS OF MISCARRIAGE

### Call your doctor immediately if

▷ You experience bleeding with cramps or pain in the center of your lower abdomen

▷ You experience pain on one side of your abdomen early in pregnancy. This could be a sign of an ectopic pregnancy (implantation of the fertilized egg somewhere other than in the uterus).

▷ Pain is severe or continues for more than one day, even if it isn't accompanied by staining or bleeding

▷ Bleeding is as heavy as a menstrual period, or light staining continues for more than three days

### Get emergency medical help immediately if

▷ You pass clots or grayish or pink material—which may mean a miscarriage has already begun. If you can't reach your doctor, go to the nearest emergency room. If possible, save the material you pass in a jar, plastic bag, or other clean container so that medical personnel can determine whether the miscarriage is threatening, complete, or incomplete and requires a D&C (dilation and curettage). In a D&C, the cervix is dilated mechanically with rods of varying sizes to allow a curette (surgical scraper) to be passed into the uterus. The curette is used to scrape off the uterine lining and the pregnancy products.

▷ You have a history of miscarriage and experience bleeding or cramping

▷ Bleeding is heavy enough to soak several sanitary pads in an hour or the pain is so severe that you can't bear it

recommendations below, the better your chances are of preventing a miscarriage.

Many women worry that an extreme movement, such as a fall, will cause them to miscarry. Miscarriages, however, are almost never caused by physical exertion, unless there is already something wrong with the pregnancy. The fetus is well cushioned and firmly attached to the inside of the womb, and it is virtually impossible for the fetus to become dislodged. Although running, jogging, and other sports have not been shown to trigger a miscarriage, low-impact exercises such as walking and swimming are considered preferable by many holistic practitioners.

# HOLISTIC APPROACHES TO COMMON FIRST-MONTH CONCERNS

The first month of pregnancy is physically and emotionally challenging. Your body switches into a *creation mode*—it begins nourishing your tiny embryo and, as a result, you may experience anxiety, nausea and vomiting (morning sickness), heartburn, or indigestion. Along with frequent urination, these are perfectly normal and may be prevented or relieved with holistic remedies.

Throughout this book, we'll give you hundreds of suggestions for preventing discomfort and keeping yourself looking and feeling terrific. During your first-month checkup, discuss with your caregiver safe holistic remedies to alleviate any symptoms or discomfort.

## Miscarriage

The following holistic remedies have been used by various practitioners to prevent early miscarriages.

### Bach Flower Remedies

English midwives have reportedly prevented miscarriages in women at risk with the *Rock Rose remedy*, which is usually taken as a tincture four times daily. There are no clinical studies on these remedies, however.

### Botanical Medicine

Canadian midwives have used *blackhaw root bark* and *false unicorn root* supplements to prevent early miscarriages in women with high-risk pregnancies. These can be taken as teas or in capsules. They should only be taken after your caregiver or herbalist has been consulted.

## Anxiety

If you're worried because this is your first pregnancy, join the club. Every pregnant woman worries. Holistic mothers worry *constructively*, however, letting it motivate them to follow all the steps outlined in this book to give themselves and their babies the best chance for a safe, natural birthing experience.

To relieve anxiety, we recommend following the holistic relaxation and exercise programs outlined in Chapters 4 and 5. You'll also find that following the healthy balanced food plan discussed in Chapter 3 and drinking soothing herbal teas of chamomile or lime-flower will also help alleviate chronic anxiety.

If you find that you have lingering worries, strike back by using the breathing, positive-thinking, yoga, meditation, visualization, and relaxation exercises described in Chapter 4. If there is a good deal of stress in your life, you may want to simplify your daily schedule to allow more time for relaxation. Also, talking to a friend or enrolling in childbirth classes can be helpful. If your anxiety persists, seek help from a counselor or psychotherapist. You may also find that some of the holistic remedies discussed below will help alleviate anxiety.

### Aromatherapy

Add two to three drops of essential oils of chamomile, lavender, bergamot, melissa, rose, or geranium to your bath water to help relieve anxiety. Alternatively, try simmering these herbs in water—making what's called an infusion—then, holding a towel over your head and a saucepan containing the boiled herbs, just inhale.

### Bach Flower Remedies

Flower remedies, such as *Rescue Remedy* or *Vervain tincture,* may help you relax and fall asleep. Bach flower remedies are often combined with psychotherapy and cranial osteopathy to help release suppressed feelings of ambivalence or fear.

### Breathing

One of the first reactions to anxiety is to hold your breath and tighten your chest. You've probably already noticed that you tend to breathe more quickly when you're anxious or worried, almost as if you're hyperventilating. Shallow, quick breathing reduces the flow of oxygen and blood to your brain—and to your baby. The following exercise will help you take your mind off worrying thoughts by focusing on your breathing.

*1.* Place your palms on the sides of your rib cage with your fingers an inch or two on either side of the sternum.

2.  Breathe in slowly and deeply to a count of three until your hands are pushed apart sideways.

3.  Breathe out slowly to a count of four or five, letting your mind focus only on your breath while you press your palms lightly against your rib cage to encourage complete exhalation.

If you repeat this breathing exercise ten to fifteen times, you'll find you're more relaxed.

You can relax anywhere, anytime, by doing this simple exercise. It's hard to be anxious when you're breathing from your belly because you're eliciting the *relaxation response*—the same set of events that occurs just before you go to sleep.

**Physical Activity**  Aerobic exercise releases *endorphins,* the body's natural pain-relieving chemicals. If you already exercise regularly, wonderful. If not, and if you're not physically limited by a chronic illness or disability, a good way to start is by walking, swimming, or bike riding at least three times a week.

**Homeopathy**  Homeopathic remedies when recommended by a homeopath are personalized, very diluted, and safe to take during pregnancy. For anxiety, especially when it is due to fatigue, ask your homeopath about taking one tablet of Aconite 6X as needed, as recommended in Dana Ullman's *Discovering Homeopathy: Medicine for the 21st Century.*

**Meditation**  Meditation is designed to help you overcome anxiety by focusing your attention on other things. The simplest type of meditation involves focusing on your breathing. Try sitting in a straight-backed chair with your back erect but relaxed. Close your eyes and pay attention to your breathing. Become aware of the soft sensations of your breath as your belly rises and falls. Try to stay focused on the complete breath: the full inhalation, the full exhalation, and the short pause in between. You may find it helpful to anchor your attention by counting each breath from one to ten (one on the inhalation, two on the exhalation, and so on up to ten).

**Shiatsu**  Shiatsu (acupressure) can also be used to relieve anxiety. Locate the shiatsu point Pericardium 6 (PC6), which is three fingerwidths above the first wrist crease on the inside of your arm. Press this point firmly for ten seconds with your thumb. Locate the same point on your other arm and press. Repeat three times.

## Depression

A lack of energy can drain you and make you feel depressed. The most common symptoms of depression include fatigue, sleep disturbances, and exaggerated mood swings caused by hormonal changes. Take a tip from women who've been there—you can turn your depression around with positive thinking.

For example, one 31-year-old first-time mother profiled in the Summer 1996 issue of *Fit Pregnancy* said she became depressed during her first month because she didn't think she could handle the responsibility of a baby. Her doctor suggested counseling, which helped. But what really lifted her spirits was a gift from a friend—a book (like this one!) that showed the month-by-month development of the baby. She suddenly started to feel positive about the changes in her body. She joined a low-impact aerobic exercise class and started jogging, walking, and biking. "My workouts gave me a sense of control over some of my body's changes," she stated. "I couldn't wait for the baby to arrive. Afterward, with exercise and a reasonable diet, I got my figure back. What's more, my relationship with my husband deepened."

The woman's recovery illustrates several key features of the holistic pregnancy program. First, information is power: the more you know about your body (and your baby's growth), the more conscientious you'll be about nutrition, exercise, relaxation, and disease prevention. So keep reading this book! Second, childbirth classes are important: you should already be thinking of joining one. Third, you have to exercise every day, because exercise will give you energy, help you sleep, make you feel good about yourself, and give you a sense of control over your body. Fourth, if you do all these things, you can replace depression and worry with positive thinking and creative problem solving. And fifth, besides preventing depression, these steps will also improve your intimacy with your partner.

Think of the momentary bouts of depression that occur during your pregnancy as little mosquitoes that bite you to remind you that you need to think positively and stay in shape.

## *Aromatherapy*

Aromatherapy acts very quickly on your nervous system and has been used to relieve temporary episodes of depression. Midwives have reported helping pregnant women recover from bouts of depression by giving them infusions of jasmine, neroli, clary sage, or rose. Two to three drops of any of these oils can be added to your bath water.

| | |
|---|---|
| *Botanical Medicines* | St. John's Wort *(Hypericum perforatum)* supplements have also been used to relieve minor depression and insomnia. Women who experience recurring bouts of depression have also reported some relief from drinking chamomile or black walnut tea. St. John's Wort capsules or tinctures and chamomile and black walnut tea are available at most health food stores. |
| *Deep-Breathing Exercises* | One of the easiest ways to prevent and relieve depression is to do quick breathing and focusing exercises throughout the day. When you're depressed, you breathe six times more rapidly than when you're not. By changing from shallow to deep breathing, you can take your mind off stressful thoughts and allow your body to relax. |
| *Exercise* | Many studies have shown that regular exercise reduces the number of depressive episodes, reduces muscle tension and anxiety, and increases self-confidence and emotional stability. Moderate aerobic activity—such as swimming, brisk walking, or jogging—may not only alleviate your depression, it may also improve your concentration, memory, and sense of self-esteem. |
| *Massage* | Just thinking about an intimate, tender massage may be enough to lift your spirits. Actually, massage has also been used effectively to treat depression, because it stimulates the release of *endorphins* (your body's natural pain killers) and reduces stress hormone (cortisol and norepinephrine) levels. It also helps alleviate insomnia, which may lead to depression. You're ahead of the game if your partner or labor coach can give you timely, effective massages throughout pregnancy and labor. We think massage is extremely important and detail several different types. Now's the time to get started—it's hard to be depressed when loving fingers are caressing you. |
| *Nutrition and Supplements* | Before you became pregnant, you were probably aware of how some foods seem to bring on minor bouts of depression. Food sensitivities and nutritional deficiencies can also cause depression. If you think your diet may be causing your depression, discuss different nutritional therapies with your caregiver. In some cases, midwives have found that adding a moderate amount of protein to the diet helps relieve symptoms without stressing the kidneys or inducing hypertension. You should also discuss the need for more carbohydrates. |

Alcohol, sugar-rich foods, soda, caffeine, and foods that contain additives such as nitrates or food colorings, as well as processed foods such as white bread, packaged macaroni dinners, canned food sauces, salami, and bologna, should also be eliminated. In addition to eating three meals daily, you might also try smaller snacks every two hours between meals until bedtime.

*Aspartame,* the artificial sweetener widely used in diet colas and foods, may be harmful to the fetus. It can also cause food allergies, sensitivities, and depression. Although according to the March of Dimes Birth Defects Foundation's *Healthy Eating During Pregnancy,* the Food and Drug Administration and the American Academy of Pediatrics Committee on Nutrition have approved aspartame as "safe for both the mother and developing baby," holistic caregivers usually advise women to avoid it during pregnancy.

Your nervous system requires an adequate supply of vitamins and minerals—including vitamins C, $B_{12}$, $B_5$ (pantothenic acid), $B_3$ (niacin), as well as folic acid, magnesium, and zinc—to function normally and avoid common neurologic and psychiatric problems, including depression. Be sure to discuss the possible need for these and other nutritional supplements with your caregiver at your monthly checkup.

## Fatigue

Don't be surprised when you suddenly have no energy. Approximately 90 percent of pregnant women suffer from fatigue during the first trimester. Fatigue is usually caused by the molecular byproducts of new cell division in the fetus and associated hormonal changes in the mother. Once the placenta is fully functional (at about twelve weeks), these biochemicals are screened out by the placenta and fatigue decreases.

Iron is an important factor in preventing fatigue, because hemoglobin (the iron-bearing compound in red blood cells) carries oxygen in the blood. Because your body cells use oxygen to create energy, an insufficient amount of iron (iron-deficiency anemia) can make you feel tired. Ask your caregiver to help you identify the causes of your fatigue, and discuss the need to add iron-rich foods (liver, red meat, fish, poultry, enriched and whole grain breads and cereals, green leafy vegetables, legumes, eggs, and dried fruit) and iron supplements to your daily diet.

| | |
|---|---|
| *Acupuncture* | One reason you feel fatigued is that your immune system may be depressed. Acupuncture can stimulate the energy channels (acupoints) that may strengthen your immune system, thereby fighting infection and eventually leaving you with more energy. It's also very relaxing! |
| *Aromatherapy* | Massage with lotions containing bergamot, geranium, or sandalwood essences mixed with almond oil has been used to overcome temporary bouts of fatigue. You can also add these essences to your bath water. |
| *Botanical Medicines* | Supplements of alfalfa, dandelion, red raspberry, and comfrey have been used to boost energy levels during pregnancy. |
| *Breathing Exercise* | Poor posture, sedentary habits, and emotional distress can result in constricted breathing, which saps your vitality, leaving you feeling dull and lethargic. The following simple exercise will help you relax and re-energize: |

1. Lie on the floor with a pillow under your knees.
2. Place your palms on your abdomen with your fingers loosely crossed just above the navel.
3. Breathe in slowly and deeply to a count of three, and feel your abdomen push your fingers toward the ceiling.
4. Breathe out to a count of four or five, while lightly pressing your palms against your abdomen to encourage complete exhalation.

Repeat this exercise ten to fifteen times.

| | |
|---|---|
| *Homeopathy* | Homeopathic remedies are frequently used to relieve anemia. Ask your homeopath about taking Ki Phos 6X three times daily to give you more energy. |
| *Nutrition and Supplements* | To increase your energy level, try switching to a diet that includes iron-rich foods, such as broccoli, egg yolks, kelp, leafy green vegetables, legumes (dry beans and peas), blackstrap molasses, parsley, prunes, and raisins. An excellent way of increasing your iron absorption is by combining these foods with foods high in vitamin C, which helps iron get in your bloodstream faster. Avoid eating bran, because it interferes with the absorption of iron into the blood. For the same reason, you should limit your intake of foods that contain oxalic acid, including |

almonds, asparagus, beets, chocolate, kale, cashews, rhubarb, soda, sorrel, spinach, and Swiss chard.

Additives found in beer, candy bars, milk and milk products (including ice cream), and soft drinks also interfere with iron absorption, as do tannins in tea, polyphenols in coffee, lead in various processed foods, and cadmium in tobacco. Coffee and tea drinkers should wait one to two hours after a meal to minimize the loss of iron. According to the U.S. Food and Drug Administration's "Caffeine Content of Food and Beverages," iron supplements are best absorbed when taken between meals, with liquids other than milk, coffee, or tea. The FDA suggests that for pregnancy, a "reasonable guideline for daily intake of caffeine is 300 milligrams"—or roughly three cups of brewed or instant coffee or five cups of brewed, instant, or iced tea. One cup of instant or brewed decaf coffee or tea contains only 2 to 3 milligrams of caffeine, so these choices are preferable. Ask your caregiver to monitor your serum iron levels to ensure that your iron intake is safe for both you and your baby.

The Institute of Medicine's *Nutrition During Pregnancy* recommends that pregnant women consume thirty milligrams of iron daily, noting that a well-balanced diet provides women a maximum of twelve to fourteen milligrams of iron. As a result, many women may need to take ferrous iron supplements. Ask your caregiver about your personal needs. Iron supplements are preferable to multivitamins containing iron, because they contain enough iron to overcome anemia. Iron supplements can sometimes mask other more serious causes of fatigue, however, such as gastrointestinal bleeding. Consult your caregiver about the proper dose of iron if you think you might be susceptible to iron overloading. Iron from natural sources is absorbed better than artificial iron, which frequently causes constipation.

## Frequent Urination

Life as a pregnant woman would be a lot easier if you didn't have to constantly go to the bathroom. As the uterus enlarges during pregnancy, it presses against the bladder, which may cause you to want to urinate more frequently. Hormonal changes, along with an increased blood volume, may also cause your kidneys to produce more urine. Because of this increased work load, the kidneys may not reabsorb sugar and protein efficiently, and these substances may spill into the urine, increasing urination.

One way to prevent embarrassing "leaks" is to lean forward when you urinate to make sure that you empty your bladder completely. If you find that you go frequently during the night, try limiting your fluid intake after 4 P.M.

*Acupressure*

The following self-massage technique has been used to help women with frequent-urination problems. Rub the acupressure point ST36 (which is two inches below the front kneecap) vigorously in a circular motion for twenty to thirty seconds. We suggest that you do this several times a day and before bedtime.

*Aromatherapy*

A mild infusion of tree oil inhaled with steamed water has been used to help reduce urinary urges. Sandalwood, bergamot, and juniper infusions have also been used to help women experiencing the urge to urinate because of infections.

## Nausea and Morning Sickness

Despite what you may have heard, you don't have to feel "sick to your stomach" throughout your pregnancy. More than 50 percent of women complain of nausea and vomiting—more popularly known as morning sickness—at some time during their pregnancy. This may be a self-fulfilling prophecy: if you think you're bound to get sick, you probably will. It's important to identify the causes of morning sickness as soon as they develop, and eliminate them.

Morning sickness (which does not occur only in the morning) is most common during the first three months of pregnancy. Excessive vomiting can cause you to lose enough fluid to become dehydrated and also develop vitamin and mineral deficiencies. Try chewing on ginger; if it's too strong for your taste, try sipping ginger tea or taking ginger supplements—they've been used effectively to relieve nausea. Eating six small meals daily, nibbling on saltine crackers in the morning, and taking vitamin $B_6$ supplements have also been proven effective.

*Aromatherapy*

Some women add essential oils of peppermint, rosewood, or chamomile to their bath water to relieve nausea. These oils have also been mixed with grapeseed or almond oil and massaged into the feet to relieve nausea. A drop of peppermint oil is also effective if taken orally on a sugar cube or as drops on the tongue.

| | |
|---|---|
| ***Botanical Medicine*** | Eating a small amount of fresh ginger has been proven an effective way of alleviating morning sickness. In a double-blind crossover trial of thirty women with nausea, twenty-five women had less severe symptoms and fewer attacks of vomiting when they took ginger supplements. In another study, ginger was more effective than Dramamine (a drug usually prescribed to prevent seasickness) in relieving nausea and vomiting. |
| ***Homeopathy*** | If you experience severe nausea that lasts more than several days, ask your homeopath about taking Ipecacuana 6X, which should be taken three times daily for five days. It can be discontinued once you notice your symptoms improving. |
| ***Nutrition and Supplements*** | Spicy and gas-producing foods contribute to morning sickness, heartburn, and belching. Some hormones may also cause acid reflux, in which stomach juices back up into the esophagus, which then becomes irritated. If you develop this condition, consult your caregiver to make sure you are not secreting too much stomach acid (hydrochloric acid). Your caregiver can then recommend an appropriate meal plan, which provides enough calories and essential nutrients for you and your baby in approximately six small meals a day. |

## Vomiting

Changes in hormone levels, diet, stress, and fatigue can result in vomiting. Consult with your caregiver to identify the causes of vomiting and to take positive steps to eliminate it.

| | |
|---|---|
| ***Acupressure*** | When you feel nauseous, apply strong thumb pressure on the inner surface of the forearm at a point two thumbwidths above the wrist crease and between the tendons. This may prevent vomiting. Seasickness bands that apply pressure to the same acupressure points can be purchased in most health stores and pharmacies. |
| ***Aromatherapy*** | Some people try to prevent vomiting by placing compresses of black pepper, chamomile, fennel, camphor, lavender, peppermint, or rose on their stomachs. These ingredients can also be used to make an infusion that is inhaled. |
| ***Nutrition and Supplements*** | We recommend a bland diet for morning sickness and to help prevent vomiting. We also recommend avoiding fried, fatty, or greasy foods; highly seasoned foods (including barbecued foods, sausage, |

and luncheon meat and other cured meats); and rich desserts such as pastries, pies, and cakes. Try to avoid large meals, and divide your daily intake into multiple small meals that you can eat every hour or two, if possible. Keep snacks—such as crackers, a plain cookie, or a piece of fruit—at your bedside so that if you wake up at night you can nibble on something. Also, try to eat something as soon as you get up and just before you go to bed. If you work outside the home, take whole grain crackers, cookies, quartered sandwiches, fruits, and celery or carrot sticks to eat on your breaks. Midwives have found that giving women vitamins $B_6$ (pyridoxine), C, and K helps reduce nausea and vomiting during pregnancy. Pyridoxine has been used to treat morning sickness since the early 1940s. Ask your caregiver to prescribe safe and effective doses of these vitamins to relieve symptoms.

*Osteopathy*

Vomiting can be caused by pressure on the cervical (neck) spine, especially at the base of the skull. This pressure is caused by the additional weight of your fetus. An osteopathic alignment can relieve this compression.

*Nutrition and Supplements*

Ask your caregiver about taking vitamin A and thiamine or acidophilus to reduce vomiting.

## Heartburn

During pregnancy, you may experience heartburn, because food moves down the digestive tract more slowly and because of the increased size of the uterus, which will begin crowding your stomach and intestines. Hormonal changes during pregnancy soften the valve (lower esophageal sphincter) between the esophagus and the stomach, allowing food and gastric acid to back up into the esophagus, irritating its lining and causing pain and an acute burning sensation in your chest. Pressure on the stomach from the growing uterus may make the symptoms worse, especially late in pregnancy. Heartburn usually occurs after meals, often as a result of eating the wrong foods or eating too quickly, but it can happen at any time, even after an emotional upset.

*Botanical Medicine*

Don't take medications to relieve heartburn, because they may not be proven safe in pregnancy. Instead of medicines such as Alka-Seltzer, antihistamines, cold pills, Di-Gel, estrogens, Gelusil, Maalox, mineral oils, Pepto-Bismol, Rolaids, Tums, or Tylenol, try taking one teaspoon of slippery elm powder mixed with one cup of water or milk. A tea made from one cup of boiled water and one cup of umeboshi plums can be flavored with tamari and drunk hot or cold to relieve symptoms. An infusion of meadowsweet may also have a soothing effect. Papaya also eases heartburn and can be consumed fresh or in tablet form. Drinking slippery elm tea or aloe vera juice is also safe and is often recommended for relieving heartburn.

*Homeopathy*

Homeopathic remedies often have bizarre names, but they're extremely effective. Taking mercurius Solubilis 6C or natrum Phosphoricum 6C three times daily, for example, relieves many cases of heartburn. These should be prescribed by your caregiver or homeopath and discontinued once your symptoms improve.

*Nutrition and Supplements*

You can also reduce symptoms of heartburn by eating frequent, smaller, low-fat meals. You should also avoid spicy, greasy, sugary, or acidic foods. Also, you should eliminate coffee and teas that contain stimulants and caffeine.

Alkaline foods, such as yogurt or milk, may also ease symptoms. For severe cases of heartburn, eating proteins and carbohydrates separately and at different times during the day may also help relieve indigestion.

# *B*IRTH SCENARIOS

In order to help you choose the caregiver and birth site that are best for you, members of this book's Medical Advisory Board have provided typical labor and birth scenarios for five different settings: a traditional hospital, an in-hospital birth center, a free-standing birth center, a home birth, and a water birth. These are for women with low-risk pregnancies, who are expecting normal births without the need for medications and with little chance of complications or emergencies. Keep in mind that hospital policies and emergencies may make your birthing experience somewhat different.

# TRADITIONAL HOSPITAL BIRTH

**First Stage:
Onset of
Labor to
Full Dilation
of Cervix**

▷ Your caregiver will let you know how strong and how frequently your contractions should occur before you and your family go to the hospital (see Chapter 10).

▷ You or your partner will be asked to fill out a registration form which will be added to your hospital file. If you're already in active labor, you may be taken directly to the labor floor.

▷ A nurse will take a brief history, asking you when your contractions started, how far apart they are, how long they last, whether your membranes have ruptured, and when you last consumed solid foods. The nurse will then check your temperature, pulse, respiratory rate, and blood pressure, and take a urine sample for analysis.

▷ Your nurse may run a fetal "test strip" via the fetal monitor, which will be attached by belts to your abdomen. Hospital policies vary on IV lines. They are usually not mandatory, so if you don't want one, discuss it with your caregiver.

▷ In a teaching hospital, a resident or intern may perform a complete physical and history and do a pelvic exam to assess effacement (thinning of the cervix), dilation, station (location of the fetus within birth canal), presentation (the part of the fetus that is pressing against the cervix when labor begins), position (relationship of the presenting part to the mother's pelvis), and pelvic capacity. In a small hospital, the obstetrician or nurse will take the history and perform the pelvic exam.

▷ The caregiver or nurse will continue to examine you periodically, as needed, to assess the progress of your labor.

▷ If your membranes still have not ruptured spontaneously and you're three to four centimeters dilated with the head engaged, the caregiver may elect to artificially rupture your membranes. Some caregivers prefer to wait until you are dilated six centimeters. Rupturing speeds up labor and allows your caregiver to determine whether or not there is meconium staining (darkened amniotic fluid). Meconium staining indicates that the baby could swallow meconium (fetal fecal matter), which could cause a serious infection.

▷ Your nurse or caregiver will also test for leaking amniotic fluid and bleeding, and monitor the fetal heartbeat with a fetoscope or a fetal monitor.

▷ Your partner may be allowed to stay in the room with you (in some hospitals, the partner will be asked to leave when you're examined). Usually you'll be allowed to suck ice chips but no other food or drink.

## Second Stage

▷ Toward the end of labor, your caregiver will examine you to verify that your cervix is fully dilated (to nine or ten centimeters).

▷ You will be taken to the delivery room, where you will be helped into a comfortable position, usually semi-sitting in your bed or on a birth stool (if you made previous arrangements to use one).

▷ Your partner will be asked to change into a scrub suit, mask, hat, and booties while you're being moved. Some hospitals allow women to deliver in the labor room, so no transfer will be needed, although your partner may still be required to change.

▷ Sterile sheets will be draped across your abdomen and legs and underneath your buttocks. Your partner may be asked to remain in the hallway while the equipment is being set up. Your perineal area will be washed with an antiseptic solution while sterile equipment and trays are prepared next to your bed.

▷ Many caregivers in traditional hospitals routinely perform episiotomies, even if you have a low-risk pregnancy and want a vaginal birth, unless you made a previous arrangement with your caregiver. Your perineum will be numbed with a local anesthetic and the cut made while you push.

▷ Once the baby's head is delivered, your caregiver will check the umbilical cord and remove excess mucus and other secretions from the baby's nose, mouth, and throat using bulb suction. In a normal birth without complications, the baby is usually full extracted on the following contraction.

▷ The baby will be placed on your stomach while the nurse clamps the umbilical cord and your partner cuts it, if he so chooses. The nurse will dry the baby, wrap the child in warm blankets, and give the child back to you to hold for several minutes.

## Third Stage

▷ The placenta (popularly called the afterbirth) usually separates from the uterus with one or two contractions and is delivered naturally, although some caregivers routinely inject Pitocin (a brand name for a hormone, oxytocin) to speed up delivery and control for bleeding. Your caregiver will administer a local anesthetic and suture any tears or episiotomy (if necessary). He or she will write orders for your care, indicating your ambulatory status (your ability to walk), foods you should be given, and pain relief and antihemorrhage medications, if needed.

## Baby Care

▷ Your baby will be checked completely within twelve hours after birth. A doctor or nurse will perform Apgar tests to evaluate your baby's development. He or she will weigh the baby; administer vitamin K and eye drops; and measure its length, head, and chest circumference. Footprints may also be taken, and your baby will get an identification tag.

▷ You will then be taken back to your room. The baby may or may not be allowed to go with you. Usually the baby is first taken to the nursery for observation and examination by a pediatrician. Your partner may not be allowed to stay in your room overnight, but visiting hours are usually fairly unrestricted.

▷ You and the baby will be examined daily, and normally you will be able to go home within two days if there are no postpartum complications.

# HOSPITAL BIRTH CENTER

## First Stage

▷ You and your family will go to the birth center when you're in active labor—that is, when contractions are three to four minutes apart and each one lasts a minute.

▷ If you've had previous care at the center, a complete physical and history may not be necessary. You and your partner will fill out consent forms and admission forms. A certified nurse-midwife or nurse will give you a vaginal exam to evaluate your progress. Your caregiver will also monitor your blood pressure and pulse, take your temperature, and take urine samples for analysis. Your baby's heart rate will be monitored by an electronic fetal monitor or fetoscope at frequent intervals. Continual fetal monitoring is not the norm, nor are test strips required for normal births.

▷ As your labor progresses, you will be encouraged to stand, sit, lie in bed, or walk around—whatever feels most comfortable. Some centers have gardens or lobbies that you can visit. You may also be encouraged to soak in a tub or take a hot shower, as hot water and pressure helps release endorphins and reduces muscle tension, thus speeding up labor. Normally, you can eat or drink whatever you choose.

▷ If there are complications such as breech position, hypertension, dark meconium staining, or slow labor, you will be transferred to the labor and delivery floor.

▷ Your caregiver will not recommend pain medications unless you ask for them, in which case you will probably be transferred to a traditional hospital birthing room.

▷ Your membranes will not be artificially ruptured. If labor is slow and your caregiver wants to speed up your contractions, he or she may induce labor, with your consent. Usually your caregiver will first try to induce contractions via nipple stimulation or acupressure, or by having you walk around. Ask your caregiver if the center will allow you to use holistic remedies, such as botanical or homeopathic medicines, Bach flower remedies, acupuncture, or hypnosis, to ease labor pains.

## Second Stage

▷ You will be re-examined once you feel the urge to push. Frequently, first-time mothers feel the urge before they are fully dilated, because the baby is low in the pelvis. You will be encouraged to push once you're fully dilated. The fetal heart rate will be taken with each contraction and your vital signs monitored at regular intervals. You will be encouraged to change positions frequently to help your baby descend. Most birth centers have birthing beds with squat bars and birthing stools that you can use. Normally you will be allowed to use pushing techniques unless your caregiver feels that your baby needs to be born sooner.

▷ Once the baby's head descends to your perineal floor, your caregiver may give you a perineal massage to stretch the perineum gently and make the passage of the head a little easier. Episiotomies are not routinely performed for low-risk births.

▷ Once the baby's head emerges, your caregiver usually will quickly bulb-suction the baby's mouth and nose to remove excess mucus, help remove the shoulders and torso, dry the baby in warm towels, and place the infant on your abdomen.

**Third Stage**

▷ Attendants at hospital birth centers allow mothers to expel placenta naturally. Breastfeeding or nipple stimulation will be encouraged to induce separation and expulsion of the placenta. If bleeding occurs or placental delivery is delayed, your caregiver may give you a Pitocin injection.

▷ Once any tears in the perineum are repaired, you will be left alone in your room with your partner and baby.

**Baby Care**

▷ A midwife or nurse will rate your baby on the Apgar scale (see Chapter 12). If the rating is not satisfactory, the baby will be given the necessary attention.

▷ A nurse-midwife, midwife, or nurse will identify your baby by taking his or her footprints and your fingerprint for hospital records and by attaching an identification band to the wrist or ankle of mother and baby.

▷ A midwife will perform the neonatal exam of the baby, recording its weight and neurological and physical signs. If required by law, your baby will be given vitamin K shots and silver nitrate eye drops to prevent infections (see Chapter 12).

▷ The nurse will diaper and swaddle the baby and give the baby back to you to nurse. You and your partner should be able to hold your baby, and you may breastfeed. The baby will be allowed to stay in the room with you and your partner overnight, if you desire.

## *F*REE-STANDING BIRTH CENTER

**First Stage**

▷ You will labor at home (see Chapter 11 for description of labor symptoms) after advising your caregiver that you've begun to labor. You will leave for the center when active labor begins.

▷ When you arrive at the birth center, you or your partner will fill out consent forms; the center should already have your pregnancy records. A nurse or midwife will monitor the fetal heartbeat with an electronic monitor or a fetoscope, assess the fetal position and stage of labor, perform the normal examinations—including blood pressure, pulse, and temperature—and take blood and urine for analysis. A pelvic exam will also be performed. Your baby will be monitored on a regular basis.

▷ If you have other children, they may be allowed to accompany you. Most centers provide gardens, kitchens, and play areas for them. Depending on your stage of labor, you will be encouraged to walk around or exercise to help advance your labor.

## Second Stage

▷ As labor progresses and transition nears, you will be encouraged to sit in a hot bath or take showers to help you relax and ease labor pains. You will be encouraged to drink high-energy liquids such as sports drinks and have snacks as long as they don't make you nauseous. Depending on the center's regulations and your caregiver's licensing, you may be offered herbal tinctures, homeopathic medicines, or Bach flower remedies to help your labor progress. Your caregiver will encourage you to change labor positions frequently.

▷ Normally, vaginal exams will be kept to a minimum. Fetal heart rate monitors are not routine.

▷ Once you're fully dilated and have an irresistible urge to push, you will be encouraged to do so. Your caregiver will continuously monitor your baby's condition and your vital signs. You will be encouraged to assume whatever positions you find most comfortable for pushing. Most centers have birthing beds, squat bars, and birthing stools.

▷ As the active phase of labor nears its end, an attendant will help your caregiver set up sterile birth and neonatal equipment close to your bed. Perineal massage is usually performed. As in all holistic births, episiotomies are reserved for emergencies.

▷ If your baby is in a breech position or other complications arise, your caregiver may determine that a cesarean delivery is necessary and you will be transferred to a hospital.

▷ Once your baby's head emerges, your caregiver eases the shoulders and torso out of the birth canal and quickly suctions excess mucus from the baby's nose, mouth, and throat.

▷ Once the baby is delivered, your caregiver or attendant will dry the baby, wrap him or her in warm towels, and place your new baby across your abdomen. The assistant will assess the baby using the

Apgar scale, then, if necessary, help you position the baby to begin breastfeeding.

▷ Once the cord has stopped pulsing, it will be clamped in two places and the father will cut it, if he so chooses. If you are Rh negative or there is a problem with the baby, the cord will be clamped and cut immediately.

## Third Stage

▷ Your caregiver will help expel the placenta naturally and then examine it for completeness.

▷ Your caregiver will suture any tears in the perineum after a local anesthetic has been administered.

## Baby Care

▷ You and your partner will be left alone to bond with the baby. Usually after thirty minutes of bonding, an attendant will perform a neonatal exam; measure your baby's length, weight, and head circumference; and give the baby a vitamin K shot and eye drops to prevent infection.

▷ If there are no complications for you or your baby, you will probably be able to return home after three to four hours. If you're advised to stay at the center, you will be allowed to stay in the same room.

▷ Upon discharge, you will be given instructions on baby care and danger signs. You will also be given your baby's birth registration papers and a postpartum checkup schedule.

# Home Births

## First Stage

▷ You will set out the supplies your caregiver has instructed you to have on hand.

▷ Your caregiver will probably arrive when contractions have been three to four minutes apart and at least sixty seconds long for one hour. If you have a history of unusually short or long latent labor, your caregiver may arrive earlier to assess you and your baby's condition.

▷ Your caregiver will encourage you to walk and stand as much as possible to increase dilation. Every thirty minutes, she will ask you to change position, if you are mainly lying down, and remind you every hour to urinate. She will also monitor your dilation, effacement, station, position, and presentation, and check your urine, blood pressure, pulse, and temperature periodically.

▷ Your baby's heart rate will be monitored frequently using an electronic stethoscope (Doppler) or a fetoscope. You will be free to use herbal tinctures, homeopathic remedies, acupuncture, Bach flower remedies, vitamin and mineral supplements, and nutritional therapies to advance your labor. Most midwives are licensed to provide holistic remedies that help ease the pain and speed up your contractions, although training and licensing vary from state to state.

▷ Your membranes will probably not be artificially ruptured, unless holistic methods are not successful in advancing labor. You will be allowed to drink electrolyte-rich liquids, such as sport drinks, between contractions.

▷ To advance your labor, your caregiver may use nipple stimulation or suggest that you take a hot shower or walk around. If your caregiver determines that you need an analgesic, a sedative, a tranquilizer, or an epidural (rarely) for pain, or if you need a cesarean delivery, you'll be transferred to a hospital.

## Second Stage

▷ Unless your labor progresses poorly or the baby's heart rate indicates the need for a quick delivery, you will be encouraged to push only when you feel like it. Your caregiver will continue to monitor the fetal heart rate.

▷ You will be advised to try a variety of pushing positions. Many home birth attendants carry a birthing stool which you may find very comfortable. Your caregiver may suggest that you try pushing while on your hands and knees, as many women find this more comfortable; in some cases, it also speeds up labor. Sometime during the second stage of labor, your caregiver's assistant will arrive and prepare sterile equipment to be placed next to your bed.

▷ Your caregiver or an assistant will give you a perineal massage when the baby's head is resting on the perineal floor. This massage significantly reduces the need for an episiotomy, and tears, if any, are normally quite small. Thus, women who have a home birth usually require no suturing.

▷ As soon as the infant's body is removed from the birth canal, the assistant will suction the nose and mouth, dry the baby in warm towels, and place your newborn on your chest or abdomen. The caregiver will then evaluate the baby using the Apgar scale and help you breastfeed—baby willing.

## Third Stage

▷ Placental delivery at a home birth can take up to one hour, because midwives prefer to wait for a natural expulsion. They will encourage you to breastfeed to stimulate your nipples; this causes your body to release its own supply of oxytocin, which increases uterine contractions and helps expel the placenta. Medications are not used routinely except to stop hemorrhaging. If there is no sign of the placenta separating after forty-five minutes, your caregiver may give you Pitocin. After that, the placenta will probably be expelled with one final push on your part.

▷ Your primary caregiver will check the placenta for fragments and completeness by inserting her hand into your uterus. This allows the caregiver to remove any remaining placental tissue and stimulates muscle contractions, which reduces hemorrhaging. She will also examine your vagina and perineum for lacerations, and suture any tears. Your caregivers will then leave you and your partner (and any friends and family you have invited) alone with the baby.

## Baby Care

▷ An hour after birth, your caregiver will return and complete the neonatal exam. Your baby will be given a vitamin K shot and silver nitrate eye drops if required or if you requested them. She will also check the baby's respiration and heart rate; measure the baby's length, weight, and head circumference; and check the baby's temperature, color, and neurological signs. Birth registration forms will be filled out.

▷ Your caregivers will probably leave about three hours following birth, after giving you instructions regarding nursing and controlling bleeding. You will be encouraged to call them if any complications develop.

▷ Your caregiver will return within twenty-four hours to examine you and the baby.

# WATER BIRTHS

**First Stage**

▷ You will begin labor at home, and go to a hospital or free-standing birth center that has a water tub when active labor begins. Unless otherwise pre-arranged, your caregiver will normally be a midwife.

▷ Your caregiver will admit you, and you and your partner will fill out registration and consent forms. Your caregiver will monitor your blood pressure, temperature, respiration, and pulse. She will also collect blood and urine samples for analysis and monitor your baby's heart rate.

▷ You will then get into the tub to relax. Your partner will be allowed to join you, if you wish. If you have good quality contractions, your caregiver will leave you and your partner alone. In early labor, you may be permitted to have a glass of wine to relax. You may also be permitted to use botanical medicines such as cohosh, as well as Bach flower remedies, aromatherapy, massage, or reflexology, to speed up contractions.

▷ As labor progresses, you will be asked to leave the tub every hour to urinate. Your caregiver will examine your vagina, checking for dilation, effacement, presentation, and position, as well as for bleeding or amniotic fluid leaks, which may indicate ruptured membranes.

▷ You will need to get out of the tub while your caregiver inspects you for meconium staining. If staining is present, you will not be able to have a water birth. In most birth centers, you will be transferred to a hospital if you have *particulate meconium* (dark green meconium) or if for any reason your labor does not progress or you need an episiotomy, medications, or a cesarean delivery.

**Second Stage**

▷ If you do not have any complications, you will re-enter the tub. You will be encouraged to push in any position you wish. Your caregiver will periodically check for effacement, position, and presentation. She will also monitor your fetus while you are in the tub, using a Doppler or fetoscope wrapped in plastic.

▷ You will begin pushing when you have the urge, usually while squatting in the tub. Your caregiver may put a squatting stool under you to assist you. Once the baby's head begins to crown, your caregiver may elevate your vagina above water to extract the baby, as this reduces the risk of infection from any contaminants in the tub. The baby will be placed on your breast, which will be out of the water, to start nursing. Once the cord stops pulsing, your caregiver will pull its loop up above the water and clamp it, and your partner will cut it.

▷ Your caregiver will quickly suction the baby's nose and mouth to remove excess mucus and wrap the baby in warm blankets. Unless there's a problem, you will be allowed to hold your baby and breastfeed.

### Third Stage

▷ Your caregiver will help you expel your placenta while you remain in the tub. You will then be helped out of the tub and given a fresh gown to put on.

### Baby Care

▷ Your baby will be given vitamin K shots and silver nitrate eye drops if required or if you requested them. Your caregiver will also check the baby's respiration and heart rate; measure the baby's length, weight, and head circumference; and check the baby's temperature, color, and neurological signs. Your baby will be evaluated using the Apgar scale, and birth registration forms will be filled out. You and your baby should be able to return home within several hours.

The first month of pregnancy is an emotional time. Sudden changes in mood are common, and you may find yourself overwhelmed by the changes in your body and emotions. The important thing is to stay confident (choosing a caregiver you trust will help enormously!) and to relax (we'll stress relaxation over and over in this book—it's the key to holistic medicine).

## Chapter 3

# The Second Month

Y THE SECOND MONTH, you no longer have any doubt that you're pregnant. By now you should feel the first signs of a tiny new human being growing inside you!

By the beginning of the fifth week of pregnancy, your baby is already one inch long and has begun to grow *fetal membranes,* called the amnion and chorion, which will form the yolk sac and umbilical cord. The umbilical cord is your baby's lifeline—oxygen, nutrients, antibodies, and hormones travel from the placenta to the fetus through the cord, and fetal waste products travel back to the placenta through the cord to enter your bloodstream for elimination.

Meanwhile, your fetus's inner layer has begun to develop three distinct layers of tissue: an outer ectoderm, a middle mesoderm, and an inner endoderm. From the *ectoderm* your baby's skin, hair, nails, parts of the teeth, plus the glands and nervous system will develop. From the *mesoderm* your baby's muscles, bones, circulatory system, and excretory system will develop. From the *endoderm* your baby's gastrointestinal tract and internal organs and glands will develop.

From the fourth week to the eight or ninth week, your baby's arms and legs develop from rudimentary buds into recognizable forms. Likewise, the eyes, ears, nostrils, and sex organs begin to form. It may seem incredible, but by the end of the second month, your baby will have a recognizable human form, with all of its systems developed.

## THE SECOND-MONTH CHECKUP

During your monthly checkups, your caregiver will check your weight and blood pressure, your baby's heartbeat, your urine, the size of your uterus, the height of the fundus, and your hands and feet for signs of edema or varicose veins. You will also be asked to describe any unusual symptoms you've been experiencing.

You probably know that during the first months of pregnancy, you will grow a whole new organ—the *placenta*—which contains blood vessels from you and your baby. The blood vessels intertwine and exchange many of the materials carried by the blood. If your nutrient stores are inadequate during the first several months of pregnancy, your baby's early development will be adversely affected—no matter how well you eat later, your baby may not recover from some of these effects.

This chapter provides many guidelines for making healthy food choices during your pregnancy. These guidelines represent the latest

### WHEN TO CALL YOUR CAREGIVER

It's important to monitor the following symptoms, which may indicate problems needing immediate attention. Although they don't always mean something is wrong, they should be discussed with your caregiver, both for your own reassurance and to guarantee that if there is a problem it is identified and treated before it progresses:

▷ Dizziness

▷ Swelling of face or fingers

▷ Severe headaches (especially frontal headaches)

▷ Vision problems, including double vision, spots in front of your eyes, or blurred vision

▷ Severe convulsions and abdominal pain

▷ Persistent vomiting after the first trimester

▷ Blood or fluid from the vagina

recommendations of leading national authorities on nutrition and obstetrics. As every woman's body is unique, however, so you should go over your personal nutritional program with your caregiver to make sure it is optimal for you and your baby.

## HOLISTIC NUTRITIONAL GUIDELINES

Imagine you have a golden vial containing a miraculous elixir that can protect both you and your baby against common medical problems. This elixir can increase your heart and lung performance, maintain your muscle and tissue strength, and even lower your body weight after childbirth.

In holistic medicine, nutrition is such an elixir, and its golden drops are the nutrients—carbohydrates, protein, fats, water, vitamins, and minerals—you need to guarantee optimum health for you and your baby. Carbohydrates, protein, and fats are relatively easy to come by in Western diets. The intake of vitamins and minerals is a little more irregular, however, because our intake of fresh fruit and vegetables is often erratic, especially among people with hectic lifestyles. The nature of these nutrients—especially vitamins—also makes it difficult to get the right amount: The *water-soluble vitamins* (B complex and C) are easily cooked out of foods because they are sensitive to heat and light; and the *fat-soluble vitamins* (A, D, E, and K) are easy to get in excess, because they are stored in the body.

### NUTRIENTS

There are six categories of nutrients present in foods: water, protein, fats, carbohydrates, vitamins, and minerals. Your body requires varying amounts of all six types of nutrients to maintain body heat, move (exertion), and build and restore bone and other body tissues.

*Water* constitutes 55 to 60 percent of an adult's body weight and is essential to life, because every cell in the body contains water. Water is needed to digest food and transport nutrients, build and repair tissues, eliminate wastes, and regulate body temperature.

*(continued)*

*(continued)*

*Proteins,* which, next to water, make up the greatest portion of human body weight, are involved in virtually every chemical process in the human body. Protein substances make up the muscles, ligaments, tendons, organs, glands, nails, hair, body fluids (except for bile and urine), enzymes, hormones, and genes. Protein is not a single, simple substance, but a complex chain of amino acids (of which there are twenty-two) that form many different chemical configurations and combine with other substances.

*Carbohydrates* are the body's chief source of energy and are also used in the synthesis of some cell components such as DNA (genetic material which makes up the chromosomes, which are found in the nucleus of each cell). An immense variety of foods, most of them derived from plants, supply carbohydrates, There are two basic types of carbohydrates: simple carbohydrates and complex carbohydrates. *Simple carbohydrates,* called sugars, include fructose, glucose (also called dextrose), and galactose, which are found alone or in combination as maltose, lactose, or sucrose (table sugar). Sugar alcohols, such as sorbitol and xylitol, are also classified as simple sugars. *Complex carbohydrates,* which are primarily starches, are large chains of glucose molecules. Starch is the storage form of carbohydrates in plants, comparable to the glycogen in humans and animals. The primary sources of complex carbohydrates are foods such as grains, bread, rice, and pasta, and starchy vegetables such as potatoes and beans.

*Fats* supply "essential" fatty acids, so called because your body cannot make them and, thus, they must be consumed in foods. Essential fatty acids help control blood pressure, blood clotting, inflammation, and other bodily functions. There are three types of fats in ordinary foods: cholesterol, saturated fats (found primarily in animal products), and unsaturated fats— either polyunsaturated fats (as found in sunflower and safflower oil) or monounsaturated fats (such as olive and canola oil).

*Fiber* is a collective term for a group of different compounds that have varied effects on the body. The most important component of fiber is *cellulose* which, although it cannot be digested, assists the digestive process. Fibers such as cellulose add bulk to the feces, thereby helping to prevent constipation and related disorders, such as hemorrhoids.

*Vitamins* are essential for important body functions such as digestion, tissue building and repair, and normal nerve functions. They also help regulate metabolism and assist in many of the biochemical processes that release energy from digested foods.

*Minerals and trace elements* are essential parts of enzymes which participate in many biochemical and physiological processes, including the transportation of oxygen to the cells. If the human body requires more than 100 milligrams daily, the substance is labeled a mineral. If the body requires less than 100 milligrams each day, the substance is labeled a trace element.

## Recommended Daily Allowances (RDA)

Most women realize that what they eat during pregnancy will impact their baby's health. But they often receive conflicting advice, which makes it difficult to develop an optimal food plan for their own health and that of their unborn child.

In order to help, the Food and Nutrition Board of the National Academy of Sciences established the Recommended Dietary Allowances (RDAs) of important vitamins and minerals that women should consume for a safe and healthy pregnancy. These are listed in Appendix D and discussed individually below.

To meet the increased RDAs for pregnancy, you must eat nutrient-rich foods and perhaps also take vitamin and mineral supplements. We strongly recommend that you try to meet as many of your nutritional requirements from foods as possible.

## Vitamin A

Vitamin A is essential for normal skeletal growth, normal immune (infection-fighting) responses, and normal night vision. In addition, vitamin A increases your ability to absorb and utilize iron. A 1993 study conducted in West Java, Indonesia, found that iron-deficiency anemia was eliminated in 97 percent of 251 women who received both vitamin A and iron pills.

Good food sources of vitamin A include meat, milk, eggs, fish-liver oils, and cheese. Leafy green vegetables (spinach, kale, bok choy, and broccoli, for example), orange vegetables (such as carrots and sweet potatoes), and yellow fruits (for example, apricots) are excellent sources of beta-carotene, a precursor molecule that the body quickly converts to vitamin A.

You should *not* take a multivitamin supplement that contains more than 5,000 international units (IUs) of vitamin A daily. A study conducted at Boston University School of Medicine found that women who took more than 10,000 IUs daily dramatically increased the risk of bearing a child with birth defects.

## B Vitamins

The B family of vitamins includes thiamine ($B_1$), riboflavin ($B_2$), niacin ($B_3$), pantothenic acid ($B_5$), pyridoxine ($B_6$), biotin, folic acid, and cyanocobalamin ($B_{12}$). The B vitamins work interdependently, so an excess intake of any one of them will generate the need for excess amounts of the others. If you're taking extra vitamin $B_6$, for example, you will need to take extra amounts of the rest of the B complex vitamins as well. These are water-soluble vitamins. Thus, excess amounts of B vitamins are normally excreted in urine—up to a point. They are also easily destroyed by too much heat or light, so careful cooking and storage procedures are essential to preserve the B vitamins in food. The different types of B vitamins are discussed below.

**Thiamine (Vitamin B₁)**

Thiamine is important for your nervous system, muscles, and heart to function normally. It also helps keep your mucous membranes—which line inner surfaces of your mouth, lungs, gut, and other organs—moist and healthy. Thiamine deficiencies are not common in pregnant women. However, a supplement is often prescribed when other B vitamins are deficient during pregnancy or breastfeeding. A thiamine deficiency may cause a loss of appetite, nervous irritability, insomnia, depression, or constipation.

Natural sources of thiamine include brewer's yeast, bran, brown rice, wheat germ, whole-grain products (such as oatmeal), beef kidney and liver, dried beans (especially garbanzo, navy, soybeans, and kidney beans), salmon, and sunflower seeds.

**Riboflavin (Vitamin B₂)**

Riboflavin is important for normal tissue growth in your fetus. It helps keep the mucous membranes healthy. It also helps decrease your craving for sugar and eases nausea and heartburn during pregnancy. A riboflavin deficiency can cause itching and burning of the eyes or cracks to develop in the skin.

Natural sources of riboflavin include milk and milk products, meats and poultry, eggs, green leafy vegetables, almonds, and brewer's yeast.

**Niacin (Vitamin B₃)**

Niacin is necessary for releasing energy from foods. It helps control fat, cholesterol, and triglycerides (fat components) levels in the blood, dilates (widens) blood vessels, and is important for normal skin and nerve function. It also promotes growth and normal digestive activity.

Natural sources of niacin include nuts, fish, dry beans and seeds, meats and poultry, brewer's yeast, whole grains, and green leafy vegetables.

Signs of niacin deficiency include inflammation of the skin, digestive disturbances, and nervous disorders characterized by muscle weakness, headaches, fatigue, depression, irritability, nausea, dizziness, and insomnia.

**Pantothenic Acid (Vitamin B₅)**

Pantothenic acid (also known as vitamin B₅) helps release energy from foods and helps build many body materials. It is found in blue cheese, brewer's yeast, corn, eggs, lentils, liver, lobster, peanuts, peas, soybeans, sunflower seeds, wheat germ, whole grain products, and meats.

There are no known deficiency symptoms for this vitamin. Nevertheless, it is usually given with other B vitamins if symptoms of any vitamin B deficiency exist, including excessive fatigue, sleep disturbances, loss of appetite, or nausea.

**Pyridoxine (Vitamin B₆)**

Pyridoxine (also known as vitamin $B_6$) is critical for the metabolism of amino acids (the building blocks of protein). When you become pregnant, vitamin $B_6$, along with niacin, helps your body absorb proteins, utilize fats, and form new red blood cells. In addition, several studies have shown that vitamin $B_6$ is also important for fetal brain development. It also helps relieve morning sickness and reduces excessive edema (abnormal swelling due to fluid retention). Consult your caregiver for appropriate dosages for each symptom.

Vitamin $B_6$ is found in avocados, bananas, bran, brewer's yeast, carrots, whole wheat flour, hazelnuts, lentils, rice, salmon, shrimp, soybeans, sunflower seeds, tuna, and wheat germ.

**Folic Acid (Vitamin B₉)**

Before the 1990s, few people had heard about folic acid or folate (also known as vitamin $B_9$). Research has shown that folic acid helps promote healthy red blood cells in both the mother and fetus. It also plays an important role in the development of a baby's nerve cells. If you do not consume adequate amounts of folic acid, you may be at risk of having a baby with *spina bifida,* a neural tube defect in which the spinal column fails to close completely. According to the American College of Obstetrics and Gynecology (ACOG), studies have shown that women who take a multivitamin containing folic acid are much less likely to have children born with neural tube defects. Other studies have shown that folate supplements can prevent almost 75 percent of neural tube birth defects if they are taken before conception or within the first two months of pregnancy. For that reason, the Food and Nutrition Board now recommends that women considering parenthood start taking folic acid six to twelve months before they try to become pregnant.

Excellent natural sources of folate include barley, beans, brewer's yeast, calves' liver, fruits, garbanzo beans (chickpeas), green leafy vegetables, lentils, orange juice, oranges, peas, rice, soybeans, sprouts, whole wheat products, and wheat germ.

The Food and Nutrition Board suggests that an easy way to consume the RDA for folate is to eat at least six servings of fortified grain foods daily in addition to five servings of fruits and vegetables. Like other B vitamins, folic acid can be partially or totally destroyed by heat and water, so cook fruits and vegetables quickly with as little water as possible. Don't throw away the folate-rich leftover water—use it in soups, sauces, or other dishes. If possible, you should consume the daily RDA for folate in whole foods. An eight-ounce glass of orange juice combined with a spinach salad at lunch and a cup of steamed broccoli at dinner, for example, supplies you with more than 300 milligrams of folate—that's three-fourths of the RDA!

### *Cyanocobalamin (Vitamin B₁₂)*

Vitamin $B_{12}$ (cyanocobalamin) helps maintain the health of all body cells, preserves nerve tissue, and enhances blood formation. It is found in animal foods such as beef and beef liver, clams, flounder, herring, liverwurst, mackerel, sardines, blue and Swiss cheese, eggs, and milk.

Strict vegetarians who do not regularly consume animal foods should take a $B_{12}$ supplement, such as nutritional yeast. Large amounts of folic acid can mask a $B_{12}$ deficiency, and large doses of vitamin C increase the need for vitamin $B_{12}$.

You need a special protein called the *intrinsic factor* to absorb vitamin $B_{12}$ from the gut. Your stomach makes intrinsic factor, but people with damage to their stomach lining (due to infection, alcoholism, etc.) don't make enough. Women who are unable to produce enough intrinsic factor may need $B_{12}$ injections. Ask your caregiver if you need to take $B_{12}$ supplements or injections.

## Vitamin C

Vitamin C (ascorbic acid) is a water-soluble vitamin that is essential for the normal development of teeth, bones, cartilage, connective tissue, and skin. It also strengthens your immune system and enhances the absorption of iron (a key component of red blood cells), thereby protecting you and your baby from infections. Along with vitamin E, it also helps prevent pregnancy-induced hypertension (PIH).

Vitamin C is present in citrus fruits, tomatoes, berries, potatoes, and dark green vegetables, such as broccoli, Brussels sprouts, collards, turnip greens, parsley, green peppers, and cabbage. Rose hips tea is also an excellent source of this vitamin.

## Vitamin D

Vitamin D is essential for healthy bones and teeth. Studies show that babies born to vitamin D-deficient mothers are more likely to have delayed formation of the top part of the skull or develop rickets. When vitamin D supplements were given in place of a placebo, however, such problems were rare.

Vitamin D is present in small amounts in milk and milk products, organ meats, fish-liver oils, and egg yolks. It is also available from the digestible bones of salmon, sardines, and herring. Vitamin D is also obtained through exposure to sunlight. Ultraviolet rays from the sun activate a form of cholesterol in the skin and convert it to a form of vitamin D, which is then absorbed by the body. Unlike the B vitamins and vitamin C, vitamin D is a fat-soluble vitamin. As a result, it is absorbed more easily in the presence of fat. Also, fat-soluble vitamins are stored in the body. Consequently, it is easy to build up an excessive amount of vitamin D in body tissues.

Ten micrograms per day, or 400 IUs, is the amount of vitamin D that is recommended to ensure the normal development of your baby. Physicians recommend that if you're pregnant and do not consume foods containing sufficient amounts of vitamin D, you should take a daily supplement. Vitamin D supplements should be taken judiciously, however, because vitamin D can accumulate in the body and cause kidney stones and kidney failure.

## Vitamin E

Vitamin E, another fat-soluble vitamin, helps promote the normal growth and development of red blood cells, nerves, and muscles. It also helps prevent damage to the lungs and to the retina of the eye. Along with vitamin C, it may help prevent pregnancy-induced hypertension.

Natural sources of vitamin E include wheat germ, liver, sunflower seeds, whole grains, walnuts, hazelnuts, almonds, butter, eggs, turnip greens, asparagus, spinach, peas, peanuts, cashews, soy lecithin, and vegetable oils.

## Calcium

Calcium is a mineral that is essential for the development of bone, and may help prevent high blood pressure in the mother. Somer's *Nutrition for Women* recommends that you consume at least 1,000 to 1,200 milligrams of calcium daily, which is the equivalent of four glasses of nonfat or low-fat milk. The RDA for calcium for pregnant women is 1,200 milligrams daily.

Calcium has also been shown to control hypertension in several clinical trials. Approximately 10 percent of American women develop high blood pressure during pregnancy, usually during the last trimester. In most cases, the elevation is mild and produces no adverse effects. However, if untreated or uncontrolled, it can progress to more serious conditions that can result in kidney failure, liver damage, seizures, and, in rare cases, death.

High blood pressure can also cause premature deliveries and low–birth-weight babies. Taking calcium supplements can help prevent these complications. A 1989 study reported in the *New England Journal of Medicine* found that only 10 percent of 600 Argentinean women who were given 2,000-milligram supplements of calcium a day during the second half of pregnancy developed high blood pressure by the time they gave birth, compared to 14.8 percent who took a placebo.

A 1992 study conducted at Brown University in Providence, Rhode Island, reported that a low calcium intake (as well as a low magnesium and potassium intake) during pregnancy increased the risk of elevated blood pressure in newborn babies. When pregnant women consumed 1,000 to 2,000 milligrams of calcium daily, however, their babies had normal blood pressures and the mothers had a lower risk for pre-eclampsia (see Chapter 6).

The best sources of calcium are milk and milk products, including yogurt and hard cheeses. Canned sardines and salmon, caviar, almonds and Brazil nuts, molasses, shrimp, soybeans, tofu, and green leafy vegetables (particularly collard and dandelion greens) are also good sources.

Calcium supplements have proved effective in maintaining recommended calcium levels. Holistic caregivers usually recommend calcium citrate capsules, because they are more easily absorbed and they reduce the risk of developing kidney stones.

Ask your caregiver to monitor your calcium levels and recommend a safe and appropriate supplement. Some calcium capsules have been reported to contain lead; others are derived from shellfish, which can trigger a dangerous reaction in sensitive people. For these reasons, questions about safety are paramount.

## Zinc

The mineral zinc is essential for many body functions. As an antioxidant, it prevents tissue damage from external and naturally occurring toxic substances. As a result, it promotes normal growth and development, aids in wound healing, enhances cell growth and repair, maintains normal levels of vitamin A in the blood, and helps synthesize DNA and RNA (the basic genetic material in body cells).

Zinc is also instrumental in many immune processes. If zinc levels are low, the concentrations of T cells (immune cells that destroy bacteria and viruses) and thymic hormones fall significantly, and many white blood cell functions critical for an immune response are severely impaired. All of these can be reversed with adequate zinc absorption.

In her book, *Nutrition for Women,* Elizabeth Somer cautions that zinc deficiency can result in congenital birth defects, low birth weight, spontaneous abortion, premature delivery, and mental retardation, as well as behavioral problems in children and an increased risk of infections and complications during pregnancy. In animals, mothers with marginal zinc deficiency produce offspring with reduced resistance to infection and disease; optimal zinc intake reverses this trend.

Natural sources of zinc include lean beef, egg yolks, fish, lamb, milk, oysters, pork, sesame and sunflower seeds, soybeans, turkey, wheat bran and germ, and whole-grain products. Diets that are high in unrefined cereals (such as granola), which contain large amounts of *phytates*—a substance that blocks zinc absorption—may result in a zinc deficiency. Studies shows that pregnant women frequently do not consume the RDA for zinc. Talk to your caregiver about ways of making sure your consumption of zinc is adequate.

## Iron

The mineral iron is essential in all cells, particularly the oxygen-carrying cells of the blood and muscles. When you become pregnant, the number of red blood cells increases 20 to 30 percent, depending on the available supply of iron. Although many practitioners recommend doubling your iron intake—from approximately eighteen milligrams a day for nonpregnant women to approximately thirty-six milligrams a day during pregnancy—most pregnant women typically increase their iron intake through foods by an average of only one to two milligrams a day. This, combined with typically marginal iron stores prior to conception, makes iron deficiency a common problem for pregnant women. Daily supplementation of thirty to sixty milligrams of elemental iron is usually recommended to prevent iron-deficiency anemia.

The dangers of iron-deficiency anemia are extensive. If you're deficient in iron, you'll be less able to tolerate blood loss during delivery and more susceptible to infection following delivery. Iron deficiency also increases the risk of spontaneous abortion (miscarriage), premature delivery, low birth weight, a stillbirth, and infant death. Infants born to mothers with anemia are at greater risk of developing anemia during their lives. You can reduce the risk of any of these complications by maintaining an adequate iron intake before and during pregnancy.

Iron is available in meats (especially organ meats), eggs, dried fruit (including raisins), fortified cereals, dried beans and peas, and dark green leafy vegetables. The iron found in animal foods is more readily absorbed than iron found in fruits, vegetables, legumes, and grains. Vitamin C makes it easier to absorb iron from these foods. Therefore, eating foods rich in vitamin C—such as citrus fruits, tomatoes, or green peppers—in the same meals can help improve iron levels in the blood.

Avoid taking iron supplements when you're consuming tea, coffee, wheat bran, or milk or milk products—these foods contain substances that slow iron absorption. Also avoid the overuse of antacids and calcium supplements, because they can also slow down iron absorption. On the other hand, iron is stored in the body and lost only through bleeding, so it's possible to accumulate too much iron in the blood. This can eventually damage the liver, pancreas, and heart. Therefore, you should not take iron supplements without your caregiver's recommendation.

## Fluorine

Fluorine helps your baby's bones and teeth grow strong by helping the body retain calcium. A small amount of fluorine, taken during pregnancy and continued throughout a baby's life, is essential for the formation of strong, decay-resistant teeth.

Although no RDA for fluorine has been established, children whose mothers consume a moderate amount during pregnancy tend to have fewer cavities than children whose mother did not get enough. On the other hand, an excessive intake of fluorine during pregnancy—that is, more than 12 parts per million (ppm) in drinking water—can produce mottled teeth in your child.

You should be able to consume adequate amounts of fluorine

from food sources, such as tea, apples, cod, eggs, kidneys, canned salmon, and sardines, and plants grown in areas where fluoride (a compound made up of two molecules of fluorine) is present in the water.

# RECOMMENDED FOOD PLAN FOR PREGNANT WOMEN

The foods you need during pregnancy are not drastically different from those provided by a normal, well-balanced diet. A variety of foods over the course of the day will provide recommended amounts of calories, protein, vitamins, minerals, and water. The guidelines below are adapted from U.S. Department of Agriculture recommendations. Individual requirements will vary; therefore, you should discuss your nutritional needs with your caregiver as soon as possible—preferably *before* you become pregnant. You may benefit from different serving

## BASIC DAILY NUTRITIONAL GUIDELINES FOR PREGNANT WOMEN

*Breads, cereals, and other whole grain and enriched products:* 6–11 servings.

One serving equals 1 slice bread; ½ hamburger bun or English muffin; 3–4 small or 2 large crackers; ½ cup cooked cereal, pasta, or rice; or 1 ounce ready-to-eat cereal.

*Fruits:* 2–4 servings (including at least one citrus fruit or juice).

One serving equals ¾ cup juice; 1 medium apple, banana, or other fruit; or ½ cup fresh, cooked, or canned fruit.

*Vegetables:* 3–5 servings (including at least two servings of dark green leafy, yellow, or orange vegetables).

One serving equals ½ cup cooked or chopped raw vegetables, or 1 cup leafy raw vegetables.

*Meat, poultry, fish, and alternative high-protein foods:* 2–3 servings.

One serving equals 6–7 ounces cooked lean meat, poultry, fish, or other protein source; 1 egg; ½ cup cooked beans; or 2 tablespoons peanut butter.

*Milk, cheese, or yogurt:* 4 servings.

One serving equals 1 cup milk or buttermilk; 8 ounces yogurt; 1½ ounces natural cheese; or 2 ounces processed cheese.

*Fats, sweets, and alcohol:* Limit fats and sweets and avoid alcoholic beverages altogether.

*Adapted from* United States Department of Agriculture Home and Garden Bulletin 232-8, 1992.

sizes, depending on your current nutritional needs, your overall fitness, and how quickly or slowly you should be gaining weight at this time in your pregnancy.

Most pregnant women will be able to satisfy the RDAs for essential vitamins and minerals by following the guidelines in the box. The USDA also suggests these additional guidelines:

▷ Limit your calories from fat to less than 30 percent of your total daily calories.

▷ Limit your calories from saturated fat to less than 10 percent of your total daily calories and your cholesterol to less than 300 milligrams per day.

▷ Eat between twenty-five and thirty-five grams of fiber each day.

▷ Try to consume about 2,000 calories of the above nutrient-dense foods a day. Check periodically with your caregiver to make sure you're getting all the calories you need, as these will vary with your body weight, your activity level, and the stage of pregnancy.

▷ Limit your calories from sugar to less than 10 percent of your daily calories.

▷ Include a vitamin/mineral supplement if your caloric intake drops below 2,000 calories. The supplement should include fluoride if your local drinking water is not fluoridated, and it should not provide much more than 100 percent of the RDA for each nutrient.

If you've already been eating a healthy diet, then moderate increases in nonfat milk products, fresh fruits and vegetables, whole grain breads and cereals, cooked dried beans and peas, fish, chicken, or extra lean meat will usually meet the increased nutrient demands of pregnancy. But if your previous diet was lacking in these foods, then you may need to make more dramatic changes in your food choices to meet your body's additional nutritional needs.

## Vegetarian Diets

A vegetarian diet is safe during pregnancy if it includes several daily servings of cooked dried beans and peas, in the same meals with whole grain foods, and low-fat milk products to meet your need for protein. If you're a strict vegetarian or vegan (who avoids all animal foods), discuss the need for supplements with your caregiver or a dietitian or nutritionist, because your diet may be low in several essential nutrients, especially protein, vitamins $B_{12}$ and D, and the minerals calcium and zinc.

Include two or more servings of dark green leafy vegetables, two or more servings of other vegetables, and one or more servings of vitamin C-rich foods each day. Six or more servings of whole grain breads and cereals (such as brown rice and oatmeal, 100 percent whole wheat bread, and whole wheat pasta) will provide trace minerals (minerals that are required in very small amounts for good health), vitamin E, fiber, some protein, and B vitamins in the daily menu. Additionally, try using one to two tablespoons of canola, rapeseed, or safflower oil (they're low in cholesterol) to make salad dressings or in cooking.

## Weight Gain

The official guidelines of the Food and Nutrition Committee of the National Academy of Sciences recommend that a woman who is at the appropriate weight for her height should gain between twenty-five and thirty-five pounds during pregnancy. Women who are underweight may need to gain more (between twenty-eight and forty pounds), and women who are overweight may need to gain less (but at least fifteen pounds) without dieting. The exercise program outlined in Chapter 5 may be helpful for obese women trying to regulate weight gain during pregnancy.

## Vitamin and Mineral Supplements

The American College of Obstetricians and Gynecologists (ACOG) guidelines on nutrition during pregnancy state that "a balanced diet that results in appropriate maternal weight gain will supply the vitamins and minerals required for pregnancy. Routine multivitamin supplementation in patients following such a diet is not necessary." If you are a healthy, low-risk woman and follow our recommended Basic Diet Plan to meet the daily RDAs for pregnancy, you probably won't need to take nutritional supplements.

Keep in mind the following exceptions. Vegetarians, according to ACOG, may need to take vitamin $B_{12}$ and zinc supplements. And mothers carrying twins or who take medications to control seizures need to take folate supplements. Vitamin D supplements, according to ACOG, are also beneficial for women who are not adequately exposed to sunlight or who do not consume milk and milk products. And some women may have to take calcium and iron supplements if they don't get the recommended RDAs in foods or they don't absorb them efficiently. The safest way to ensure that you do not have to take supplements is by having your nutritional intake evaluated at each monthly checkup.

## Junk Food

You need to avoid junk food in which calories are supplied mainly by sugar and fat. Limit candy, potato chips, and other commercial snack foods, pastries, desserts, and soft drinks until only after you've satisfied your nutrient requirements each day. It's also best to avoid artificial sweeteners, because their effects on pregnant and lactating women have not been fully studied.

### Salt

Salt is a compound made of two elements: sodium and chloride. *Sodium* is of concern for people with high blood pressure, because it helps keep fluid in the body, thereby raising the total fluid volume and blood pressure. Your sodium requirements during pregnancy increase slightly, so salt is not prohibited. But most Americans already consume more sodium than they need from the foods they eat. So, you probably won't need to add salt to your diet.

At one time, salt was routinely restricted during pregnancy to reduce the risk of *toxemia* (hypertension combined with fluid retention and protein in the urine). According to the International Food Information Council Foundation's booklet, *Healthy Eating During Pregnancy,* the latest studies show that there is "no evidence that sodium restriction prevents or alleviates toxemia."

Some pregnant women may be genetically at risk for developing hypertension and toxemia. If you have a family history of high blood pressure, discuss with your caregiver the need to restrict your salt intake while you're pregnant. It's a good idea for all women to identify a safe and healthy sodium level as early in pregnancy as possible. If for any reason you need to reduce your salt intake, ask your caregiver about taking herbal salt substitutes, which are safe for salt-sensitive people.

### Sugar

Sugar is not necessarily an unhealthy food, but it does provide calories without providing nutrients. Researchers do not agree on the maximum amount of sugar that is safe for pregnant women. Again, the best advice is to discuss this with your caregiver.

## Caffeine, Alcohol, Cigarettes, and Drugs

### Caffeine

According to the International Food Information Council's booklet, *Healthy Eating During Pregnancy,* contradictory research findings have been reported on the effects of caffeine during pregnancy. A 1993 study by the National Institutes of Health (NIH) found that pregnant women who consumed as many as three eight-ounce cups of coffee, seven-and-one-half eight-ounce cups of tea, or five twelve-ounce cans of cola did not have a greater risk of miscarriage or delivering a low–birth-weight baby than those who avoided caffeine. Fueling the caffeine controversy, however, was another 1993 study of 1,324 women conducted by McGill University in Montreal, which found that pregnant women who consumed the amount of caffeine in one-and-one-half to three cups of coffee a day nearly doubled their risk of miscarriage. This risk was tripled when more than three cups of coffee a day were consumed.

Although the FDA has stated that "there is insufficient evidence to conclude that caffeine adversely affects reproduction in humans," the best advice is to have as little as possible. The NIH suggests a maximum daily caffeine consumption of 300 milligrams. A five-ounce cup of brewed (by drip method) coffee contains approximately 115 milligrams of caffeine, a five-ounce cup of iced dark tea contains 60 milligrams, most six-ounce soft drinks contain about 18 milligrams, an ounce of Baker's chocolate contains 23 milligrams, an ounce of dark semi-sweet chocolate contains about 20 milligrams, and an ounce of milk chocolate contains about 6 milligrams. If you must drink coffee, try limiting your intake to two cups daily and avoid medications that contain caffeine. Better yet, try decaffeinated coffee and caffeine-free teas and sodas that are available at your grocery store or health food store.

### Alcohol

Health authorities recommend not drinking alcohol at all during pregnancy.

Although alcohol consumption is most dangerous during the first trimester and, in some cases, varies with the woman's size and health status, holistic caregivers also recommend that you not drink alcohol throughout your entire pregnancy. The U.S. National Institute of Alcohol Abuse and Alcoholism cautions that three or four beers or glasses of wine a day may cause mental retardation, hyperactivity, a heart murmur, or facial deformities, such as a small head or low-set ears. In some clinical studies, alcohol has been shown to slow the growth of the developing infant and result in irreversible problems that appear at birth or months to years later—a condition called *fetal alcohol syndrome.* Thus, the safest recommendation we can make is to avoid all alcohol just before and during pregnancy.

**Smoking**

Most research indicates that pregnant women should not smoke during pregnancy. The National Center for Health Statistics, for example, reports that pregnant women who smoke are much more likely to have problem pregnancies and low–birth-weight babies. Among white women, 9.4 percent of those who smoked during pregnancy had babies who weighed less than five pounds eight ounces, compared with 4.8 percent of nonsmokers. Among black women, the rate of low birth weight for babies born to smokers was 21.2 percent, compared with 11.7 percent for babies born to nonsmokers.

Cigarette smoking also reduces the amount of oxygen available in your blood supply, which directly affects the growth of fetal tissue. According to recent studies, babies born to mothers who smoke thirteen or more high-tar cigarettes a day during pregnancy are smaller and in worse physical condition than those born to nonsmoking women. In addition, German researchers have found that smoking just one cigarette a day raises the heart rate in both the mother and fetus. Smoking also promotes growth retardation in infants born to some women with pregnancy-induced hypertension (PIH). In light of increasing evidence that smoking or secondhand smoke is harmful to both you and your baby, you should be extremely careful about not smoking and strictly limit your exposure to tobacco smoke. If your partner smokes, he should stop, or at least not smoke in your presence.

**Recreational Drugs**

You must avoid all recreational drugs during pregnancy. Marijuana has not been conclusively proven to cause birth defects, but the extended inhalation that is typical among marijuana smokers allows even more tar and carbon monoxide to enter the lungs than does regular cigarette smoking.

Cocaine and opiates are among the most dangerous recreational drugs for pregnant women. According to the ACOG's bulletin, *Screening for Drug Abuse,* these drugs are associated with poor weight gain during pregnancy, impaired fetal growth, and an increased risk of premature birth and *abruptio placenta* (early separation of a placenta from the uterus; see Chapter 10). Cocaine may also cause certain congenital defects, although according to ACOG, proof of this has not been firmly established. Babies born to women who used cocaine also exhibit withdrawal symptoms, such as tremors and hyperexcitability.

*Prescription Medications*

Some medications can cross the placenta and adversely affect your fetus. They may also pass through your breast milk. Talk to your caregiver before taking any prescribed medications. It may be necessary to stop breastfeeding until all prescription drugs have passed out of your system.

*Aspirin*

At one time, aspirin was thought to decrease high blood pressure during pregnancy in certain women who were already at high risk for PIH. As a result, some caregivers began recommending low doses of aspirin for patients at moderate or low risk, based on the theory that it might help and was probably not harmful. Other studies have found little benefit in giving aspirin routinely to healthy pregnant women as a way of preventing high blood pressure. Talk with your caregiver before taking aspirin, because it can prolong bleeding. In small doses, it may be safe and effective when taken under supervision.

## Holistic Approaches to Common Second-Month Concerns

Flatulence and constipation are common during the second month, and they can be irritating. Here are several holistic approaches to prevent or relieve them.

### Flatulence

Beginning in the your first month, you may experience flatulence (intestinal gas), which is formed by the fermentation of material in your gut by the bacteria that normally reside there. It may also occur in women who cannot digest certain carbohydrates (such as *lactose*— the natural sugar in milk) and other foodstuffs, who swallow air, or develop constipation. It can also be caused by an excessive intake of B vitamins and iron supplements. The symptoms include abdominal discomfort and/or chest pains which may be mild and feel like slight pressure.

Flatulence caused by constipation can be relieved by drinking more fluids. Ask your caregiver to evaluate your B vitamin and iron intake and to prescribe appropriate doses that will fulfill your nutritional requirements and ease your symptoms.

*Aromatherapy*

Midwives have found that inhaling infusions of bergamot, chamomile, fennel, juniper, lavender, peppermint, rosemary, or coriander oil helps relieve flatulence. Add a teaspoon of any of these oils to a quart of boiling water and inhale the vapors. There are no clinical trials on the effectiveness of these oils.

# ESPECIALLY *for* FATHERS

YOUR PARTNER'S PHYSICAL AND EMOTIONAL CHANGES will affect her eating, sleeping, and work routines and her sexual desire—and they'll affect yours as well. These changes are normal, but may be uncomfortable for her. Make a special effort to familiarize yourself with the holistic practices in this book, which may help you avoid or resolve these problems. You're a key part of her holistic pregnancy team! Your moral support—not to mention your back rubs and massages—can prevent a lot of aches and pains and do wonders for her spirit—and your baby's!

Because of changes in hormone levels, it's normal for a woman's sex drive to change during pregnancy. Your sexual desire may also change as her pregnancy progresses. Being honest with each other about your needs and emotions is the key to a satisfying sexual relationship during and after pregnancy.

You may wonder if intercourse will harm the baby or your partner. In a low-risk pregnancy, sex is considered safe and healthy up to shortly before the baby is born. Your partner's comfort should be the most important guide to sexual activity. You may wish to use positions that don't put pressure on her abdomen, such as lying on your sides together or with you lying underneath.

If your partner does have health problems, ask your caregiver whether sex will be safe. You may be advised to modify your lovemaking, to use a condom, or to abstain from intercourse for the health of your partner or the baby. If your partner develops any problems—such as bleeding or contractions—during the sex act, call her caregiver right away.

**Botanical Medicine**

Flatulence may also be relieved by adding a teaspoon or two of superfine white, green, or yellow French clay (similar to bentonite) to a cup of spring water. Drink the mixture at least once a day after meals. The clay absorbs the impurities and gas with no reported side effects.

An alternate therapy is to drink a tea made from a teaspoon of anise seeds added to a cup of water. Flatulence has also been relieved by coffee enemas, which help the kidneys eliminate toxins.

**Nutrition and Supplements**

Blander foods and smaller meals may help reduce flatulence. Chewing your food more slowly and thoroughly and eating more high-fiber foods may also help. Identify and avoid foods that may cause intolerant or allergic reactions. You may also try to avoid protein- and carbohydrate-rich foods together in the same meal. Some midwives recommend chewing parsley sprigs after meals or sipping diluted lemon juice or apple cider vinegar with meals. Others suggest adding more fermented products—such as yogurt, kefir, and buttermilk—to your diet.

Ask your caregiver if you should take supplements such as vitamin B complex, acidophilus, charcoal tablets, peppermint oil, or aloe vera juice to relieve flatulence.

## Constipation

Virtually every woman (especially women who are overweight) experiences constipation during pregnancy. Functional changes in your intestines as well as the pressure of your expanding uterus on the lower bowel and rectum can produce constipation. Furthermore, the combination of constipation and increased rectal pressure puts you at risk for hemorrhoids and may produce rectal burning.

The best way to prevent constipation or its effects is to follow a high-fiber diet and exercise regularly. Physicians also normally advise women to drink at least eight to twelve glasses of water every day; to eat four to six servings of fresh fruits, vegetables, and whole grains daily; and to increase their level of physical activity. Avoid taking laxatives, too, unless they are recommended by your physician.

**Acupressure and Acupuncture**

You can relieve constipation with acupressure by pressing firmly against acupuncture point CV6 which is three finger widths below the belly button and between your navel and your pubic bone. Gradually press in one inch deep, and maintain this pressure for three minutes while breathing deeply and keeping your eyes closed.

Acupuncture may also restore the natural peristaltic (wavelike) action of the colon and alleviate constipation. Acupuncture treatments are often supplemented with rhubarb root, aloe vera, and senna leaves taken as a tea.

### Ayurvedic Medicine

An Ayurvedic remedy that has been recommended to relieve constipation consists of drinking one cup of hot milk (nonfat or low fat) mixed with a teaspoon of ghee (clarified butter) before bedtime. This acts as a mild laxative. An alternative is almond oil with a dash of sugar added; this increases *peristalsis* (wavelike contractions of muscles in the intestinal wall that help push food along the intestinal tract). It's also important to make sure your diet contains enough fiber. Beets and cabbage are excellent for women who find that bran-rich foods, such as wheat or oat bran, are too harsh or who tend to be anemic and should therefore limit their intake of bran.

### Botanical Medicine

Cascara (buckthorn) supplements can also relieve constipation by increasing peristalsis. Cassia senna leaves and psyllium seed husks have the same effect. A typical dose consists of one to two rounded teaspoons of cassia senna leaves or psyllium seed husks stirred in eight ounces of water after meals. A half teaspoon of *Lactobacillus acidophilus* with an eighth of a teaspoon of *Bifidobacteria bifidum,* taken twenty minutes before meals each day, will also relieve constipation.

### Exercise

Exercise helps stimulate muscle contractions in the colon. One of the safest and most effective exercises for relieving constipation is brisk walking.

### Bowel Exercises

Sometimes constipation occurs because people ignore their body's signal to empty their bowels. It's a good idea to set aside time in the mornings and after meals for the purpose of having a bowel movement. The urge to defecate is partially beyond conscious control, but training yourself to have bowel movements at regular intervals helps encourage the body to eliminate wastes.

### Homeopathic Medicine

Ask your homeopath about taking Nux Vomica 6X three times daily to relieve mild constipation.

### Hydrotherapy

Taking a cool, five-minute sitz (sitting) bath may relieve minor constipation. Alternatively, try a cold compress on your forehead and a glass of cold water. Alternating hot and cold showers may also be effective. For chronic constipation, place a cold compress covered with a large, dry towel on your abdomen.

**Mild Laxatives**

It's safe to use mild, natural laxatives such as milk of magnesia during your pregnancy. You can also try a glycerine enema, which is available in disposable packages at most drugstores.

**Nutrition and Supplements**

The two Fs, fluids and fiber, are essential for reversing constipation. Feces are composed primarily of water, so drinking lots of water will help ensure softer, easier-to-eliminate stools. If you experience continual constipation, try drinking ten glasses of water a day. Bran fiber is also excellent for relieving constipation because it produces a softer stool. Raw bran (with large particles) is more effective than processed bran. "Bran therapy" should be short term, however, because too much bran can rob your body of essential nutrients, especially iron. Ask your nutritionist how much bran is safe to take to relieve constipation and how long you should take it.

Vitamin C supplements, evening primrose oil, and folic acid supplements have been used to relieve constipation. Ask your caregiver if you should add these supplements to your current vitamin and mineral regimen.

Iron supplements may produce constipation. Ask your caregiver for tips on meeting the RDA for iron without supplements or with a different formulation.

## Other First-Trimester Concerns

Don't be surprised if you wake up in the middle of the night craving pickles. Unusual food cravings are caused by hormonal changes and are quite common in pregnancy. They are usually harmless, and it may be less stressful to indulge an occasional craving than to deny them, as long as you continue to consume the recommended number of servings of foods that meet the RDAs for essential nutrients.

Some women develop rather bizarre cravings for chalk, clay, or laundry starch. Such cravings are called *pica*. If you develop persistent, bizarre cravings, discuss them with your caregiver.

And don't be alarmed if you suddenly find yourself sweating! Sweating is your body's way of cooling itself. Your body temperature rises when it burns food for energy. The process of "burning" is called *metabolism*. The higher your *metabolic rate,* the more heat is produced and the more likely you are to sweat. Your basal metabolic rate (the rate at which food is burned to meet all energy needs except the energy for physical activity) will increase by 20 percent during pregnancy, and one result is that you feel overheated and sweat more. You'll perspire more, particularly at night. Although sweating is beneficial because it helps to cool you off and rids your body of waste products, it can be unpleasant. To minimize any discomfort, bathe often, and use a good antiperspirant and/or powder. And dress in layers—especially in winter. This will allow perspiration to escape from the layer of clothing nearest your skin. It will also let you peel down to shirtsleeves when you start heating up. Remember to drink extra fluid to replace the fluid lost through sweating.

When two expectant mothers meet in a caregiver's office, the first topics of conversation are usually weight gain and nutrition. "What foods are you eating? How much weight are you planning to gain? How much have you gained so far?" Hopefully, having read this chapter, you've already developed the best holistic food plan for your health, lifestyle, and tastes. This diet will give you lots of energy—which you'll need for the holistic exercise program described in the next chapter.

## Chapter 4

# The Third Month

*E*VERY DAY YOUR LITTLE MIRACLE continues to grow!
It's probably still hard for you to imagine that there's a living, growing baby inside you. But by now your baby is two to three inches long and weighs about half an ounce. Its circulatory and urinary systems are functioning, its liver is producing bile, and its reproductive organs are developed. Also, its heart is beating, and it can move its arms and legs—a result of both muscle and nerve development.

Several important changes will take place inside your body this month due to changes in the activity of *progesterone,* the female sex hormone that sustains your pregnancy. Until now, this hormone has been secreted almost entirely by the *corpus luteum,* a small body of cells in the ovary, which formerly contained the ovum (egg) that is now the fetus growing inside you. The corpus luteum produces both female sex hormones: progesterone and estrogen. It starts to shrink about six or seven weeks after the last menstrual period and shuts down completely at about ten weeks. During its three to four weeks of operation, its hormones promote the growth and development of the uterus to ensure successful implantation. Once the corpus luteum shuts down, the uterus starts producing progesterone. Because this hormone tends to relax smooth muscle tissue, muscle contractions along the gastrointestinal (GI) tract become weaker and food moves more slowly through your system, resulting in bloating and indigestion.

Your blood pressure will increase slightly, because you're now pumping more blood to the growing fetus. This can cause fatigue, dizzy spells, and headaches.

One way to offset these and other symptoms is to follow the Holistic Exercise Program outlined in this chapter. The exercises may help prevent or relieve constipation, fatigue, bloating, and swelling.

# ESPECIALLY *for* FATHERS

DON'T BE SURPRISED if you find that you sometimes have mixed feelings about your partner's pregnancy. You may wonder if you can meet the financial and emotional responsibilities of raising a child. And you may get frustrated by the day-to-day change in your household routine. You may also be concerned about how pregnancy and a child will change your life and your relationship with your partner.

These feelings are *normal*. Being honest with yourself and talking openly with your partner can increase your intimacy and ensure the best possible outcome for the baby. Early pregnancy is an emotional time for your partner. Sudden changes in mood are common, and she may focus her thoughts inward. Mixed feelings are common for you, too, as you become more concerned about your partner's health. The best thing you can do is to understand the physical and psychological changes that both of you are experiencing and try whatever methods are available.

One intimacy exercise you can try is to sit down every evening and meditate together. Start by doing a breathing exercise (see Chapter 5), then look into each other's eyes without speaking for several moments. Next, begin taking turns telling each other how you feel physically and emotionally. Let your partner speak while you listen without commenting. Being good listeners, sensitive to each other's needs, will enhance communication and help both of you meet your challenges in a calm manner.

This is also a good time for both of you to recommit yourselves to a lifestyle that will ensure a healthy childbirth. Help your partner plan a balanced, holistic food plan; exercise with her if you can; get plenty of sleep; and avoid alcohol, tobacco, and other drugs. Working together will benefit you, your partner, and your baby.

They'll also increase your muscle tone, strength, and endurance, which will make it a lot easier for you to cope with the physical stress of pregnancy and labor. The most important benefit is that they'll increase your feelings of self-control and self-esteem.

## THE THIRD-MONTH CHECKUP

This month's checkup is the ideal time to review your personal exercise program. You may want to consider adding exercises in the Holistic Exercise Program described in this chapter. Ask your caregiver if you have any medical conditions that could require you to modify your exercise routine.

Fatigue, dizzy spells, and headaches are also common during this month. Several holistic remedies that have been used to resolve these problems are detailed in this chapter. Feel free to discuss them with your caregiver. Remember: you and your caregiver are partners in the miracle of childbirth—the more communication between you, the better.

## HOLISTIC EXERCISE PROGRAM FOR PREGNANCY

Let's be honest: The idea that exercise can make labor easier should be enough to motivate you to indulge in some form of safe physical activity every day. ACOG's *Exercise During Pregnancy and the Postpartum Period* describes a study of 845 pregnant women by researchers at the University of Florida who found that women with low-risk pregnancies who did aerobic exercises—such as riding a stationary bike and weight lifting—three times a week had shorter hospital stays and fewer cesarean deliveries than women who did not exercise. Another study by Case Western Reserve University in Cleveland found that physically fit women who continued to exercise during pregnancy used approximately half as much pain medication as women who did not exercise and that women who exercised right up until delivery experienced shorter labors than women who quit exercising!

These studies strongly suggest that regular exercise is vital for women with a low-risk pregnancy. Those with complications—such as a threatening miscarriage, diabetes, or PIH—may be advised by their caregiver to stay in bed intermittently.

# PHYSICAL ACTIVITY RECOMMENDATIONS OF THE AMERICAN COLLEGE OF OBSTETRICIANS AND GYNECOLOGISTS (ACOG)

According to recent ACOG guidelines, physical fitness and active recreation will enhance your self-esteem and sense of well-being during pregnancy. The guidelines stress that there is "no point in exercising strenuously, since a pregnant woman can maintain cardiovascular fitness through mild to moderate exercise." *Strenuous exercise* is defined as "an exercise level during which a woman cannot converse normally." ACOG suggests that the intensity of all exercises should be reduced gradually during the last trimester.

ACOG has the following specific recommendations:

▷ Avoid contact sports that could result in abdominal injury.

▷ Try swimming and water aerobics (provided the water is neither too warm nor too cold); these may be the best forms of exercise immediately prior to childbirth, because water supports your weight and allows you to work out vigorously throughout pregnancy. The ACOG guidelines caution that you should monitor your body temperature while exercising and avoid overheating.

▷ Stop exercising if you develop any of the following symptoms:

— breathlessness
— dizziness
— muscle weakness
— nausea
— chest pain or tightness
— back, hip, or pubic pains
— vaginal bleeding
— leakage of amniotic fluid
— difficulty walking
— a racing heart while resting
— uterine contractions
— changes in fetal movement

Women who were sedentary before becoming pregnant should start with very low-intensity activities and build up gradually.

## Pregnant Women Who Should Not Exercise

ACOG suggests that women with the following medical conditions should not exercise during pregnancy:

▷ pregnancy-induced hypertension (PIH)

▷ history of premature labor

▷ persistent bleeding

▷ incompetent cervix

▷ retarded fetal growth, as determined by sonography

▷ premature rupture of the membranes

Women with chronic medical conditions, such as cardiovascular or pulmonary disease, should first be evaluated by their physician to determine what kind of exercise, if any, is suitable.

## Getting Started

Now that you know it's important to exercise, it's time to get started. To help you begin, we have put together a simple program of eighteen exercises that combine swimming, walking, aerobics, Kegel exercises, towel exercises, yoga, calisthenics, and weight lifting. This comprehensive exercise program is designed to tone your entire body, not just your pelvic muscles. To keep you from getting bored, we've made each day's exercise routine different.

The upper-body and abdominal exercises will help improve your posture while you gain weight. The cardiovascular exercises will increase your endurance and stamina to help make childbirth a little easier. The stretching exercises will protect your joints, muscles, and connective tissues from injury during physical activity, weight gain, and childbirth. All of the exercises are recommended by midwives as safe and effective.

We encourage you to develop your own wellness program by integrating these movement exercises with the relaxation and breathing exercises described in Chapter 5. You can do simple exercises first thing in the morning, right before bed, or during a coffee break. Psychologically, it may help if your partner does these exercises with you. When you begin the program, you may experience some muscle soreness and fatigue—especially if you haven't been exercising on a regular basis. But if you stick with our Holistic Exercise Program, the time you spend exercising will soon be repaid in the energy you gain every day.

## Aerobic Exercise

*Aerobic exercise* is continuous activity that raises your heart rate. Its benefits are well known. Low-impact aerobic activities—such as walking, swimming, stair climbing, and stationary cycling—safely stimulate your heart and lungs and help increase your ability to use oxygen, which is a plus for you and your baby. Remember: you're exercising too much if you cannot carry on a normal conversation.

### *Aerobic Dancing*

Aerobic dancing does the same great stuff as running, swimming, or any good workout. It strengthens your heart and other muscles, helps burn body fat, lowers blood pressure and cholesterol, helps control heart disease, boosts "brain power" (people who exercise regularly have quicker mental reaction times and better memory and reasoning abilities), improves your sex life (by increasing stamina), and helps reduce pain by releasing endorphins.

Unlike the loneliness of long-distance running, aerobic dance is a social activity. And, unlike a swimmer or bicyclist, you don't have to worry about weather conditions or buying expensive equipment—a good pair of sneakers will do. You don't even have to be athletically inclined. In short, it's fun and inexpensive, and you can do it at home while watching video tapes or, even better, with a friend or two.

*Swimming*

When the added weight of your baby shifts your center of gravity, swimming in a warm pool is the safest and most comfortable form of aerobic exercise. It allows you to safely maintain your cardiovascular fitness throughout your entire pregnancy. Also, it will not over-stress your legs and you won't perspire or become overheated. Most women are able to swim until the day they deliver.

*Walking*

It doesn't come in a bottle, it's not a pill—and it's absolutely free. Walking is a "miracle exercise" that is often forgotten. It is a potent therapy—it helps prevent heart disease and diabetes, lowers blood pressure, reduces anxiety, relieves back pain, strengthens your immune system, and enhances your self-esteem and your social life. It can make you feel more energetic and less stressed while controlling your weight; preventing insomnia, varicose veins, and swollen ankles; and, best of all, improving your sex life.

Walking briskly for 20 to 45 minutes three times a week is a good cardiovascular workout. Be sure to buy good supportive shoes designed for walking.

*Social Dancing*

Do you want to build cardiovascular fitness and add romance to your relationship? Try social dancing once a week. It's not just the heart-strings that get pulled by a good fox-trot: the heart itself gets a healthy push. Studies show that the cha-cha, polka, samba, waltz, and swing dancing can raise the average person's heart rate enough to achieve an aerobic conditioning effect.

*Gardening*

Think of it as your own private health club—an invigorating fresh-air gym replete with body-building equipment, aerobic sessions, resistance training—and an occasional squirrel. Where else but in a garden can you pump your pectorals amid the petunias and tone your biceps in a turnip patch? All the equipment you need is a spade, a wheelbarrow—and a one-pound sack of topsoil.

Gardening takes you through a wide range of physical movements and works almost every muscle in your body. Not only do you tone your muscles when you garden, but you keep those extra pounds from adding on too fast as well. The continuous action of raking, hoeing, and digging burns almost as many calories as a moderate aerobic dance workout—almost 300 calories an hour. Studies show that gardening activities lower your risk for a number of health problems, including high blood pressure, diabetes, and heart disease. If you choose gardening for your exercise routine, be sure to wear gloves, long-sleeved shirts, and long pants to protect against contaminants such as herbicides, insecticides, and cat feces.

*Stair Climbing*

The stair-climbing machine gives one of the best high-intensity, low-impact workouts. It's safe, you can control the intensity of the workout, and it's fast! It can deliver an aerobic workout in twenty minutes. It provides an excellent lower-body workout, exercising large muscle groups in the legs and lower back. It's also excellent for your postpartum recovery, because it helps you rebuild your lower back strength and improves your gait, balance, and functional mobility. And because your bones bear weight during stair climbing, it helps build stronger bones without putting your musculoskeletal system at risk.

## Kegel Exercises

In the 1950s, Arnold Kegel, a professor at the University of California at Los Angeles, observed that the majority of women who had complications after pregnancy had not exercised regularly during pregnancy. He designed a series of gentle exercises that strengthen the vaginal, urethral, and anal muscles. We recommend that you do Kegel exercises every day in either a seated or standing position during pregnancy, and for the rest of your life.

Kegel exercises are contractions of the pelvic floor, or *perineum* (the sheet of muscles located at the base of the pelvis which supports the pelvic organs). Kegel exercises help prevent incontinence and abdominal, pelvic, vaginal, and urethral pain during pregnancy. Doing them regularly will also lessen the risk of vaginal tearing and the need for an episiotomy. Following birth, Kegel exercises will help strengthen your pelvic floor muscles, increase nerve activity and blood circulation in the sex organs, and prevent postpartum incontinence.

## KEEP EXERCISING

Thinking about exercise is a lot easier than doing it. Here are several hints to get you started:

1. *Make the decision.* Your well-being—and that of your baby—depends on your exercise routine. If you stop exercising, you'll start to lose some of your energy, longevity, and creativity. Remember: You're exercising for two—you can't afford not to give your baby the best start in life.

2. *Set goals.* Goals act as psychological magnifying lenses, focusing your efforts to pick a good program and reinforcing your energy during each workout. Studies show that people who exercise and set *specific* and *challenging* goals— such as adding ten minutes to their program each week—are more likely to achieve them and consistently outperform their procrastinating peers.

3. *Reward yourself.* People don't quit activities that are fun. Reward yourself each time you accomplish an exercise objective. One little word of advice: *Don't use food as a reward.* Somewhere down the line, this reward will turn on you. Find a reward that's almost as much fun—treat yourself to a bubble bath, a movie, or a good book.

4. *Cross train.* Alternate your exercises each day—running one day, then lifting weights, gardening, or practicing martial arts another.

5. *Keep your dates.* In one study, almost half the subjects quit because they said they didn't have time. You have to *make* time.

6. *Count the benefits.* When things get tough—your legs ache, for example— remind yourself that you're exercising for two. Improving the quality of your life and your baby's life makes it all worthwhile.

You also can use Kegel exercises to enhance sexual pleasure for yourself and your partner, as they help create a "tighter vaginal fit" which increases friction. Within a few weeks, you should be able to increase the amount of time you're able to hold contractions and the number of repetitions you're able to complete. Your goal should be to work up to ten-second contractions, followed by ten seconds of relaxation, and to complete as many repetitions as you can.

In the beginning, check yourself frequently by looking in the mirror or by placing a hand on your abdomen and buttocks to make sure that you do not feel your belly, thigh, or buttock muscles move. There should be no visible movement while doing Kegel exercises.

**Standing Kegel Exercise**

If you don't know where the pelvic floor muscles are, sit on a toilet and try stopping and starting your urine flow. Those are the muscles you want to be contracting. Now that you know which muscles you're exercising, here's how you work them:

1.  While standing, imagine pulling a pencil into your vagina. This will tighten your pelvic floor muscles, pulling them upward and inward toward your body's midline.

2.  Maintain the contraction for six seconds, then relax the muscles.

    Kegels may also be done on the toilet; in fact, they're best performed after urinating. Do six Kegels each time you finish urinating, throughout your pregnancy.

**Lying-Down Kegel Exercise**

1.  Lie on your back with your knees bent, your feet about twelve inches apart, and the soles of your feet flat on the floor. Your head and shoulders should be supported by cushions and your arms resting against your sides.

2.  Firmly tense the perineal muscles (if you don't know where they are, read the description under *Standing Kegel Exercise,* above). Hold for as long as you can (eight to ten seconds), then slowly release the muscles and relax.

3.  Do at least twenty-five repetitions at various times during the day.

    You can also do this exercise while urinating or at your desk at work, driving in the car, or standing in line at the grocery store. Kegels can be done virtually anywhere.

## Towel Exercises

An easy exercise you can do at home involves using your body weight as a natural form of resistance to slowly and gently stretch your muscles with a controlled range of motion. A towel is used to help keep your back in alignment while you exercise.

We recommend that you do the towel exercise at least twenty minutes a day in addition to relaxation exercises, walking, swimming, or yoga. Hold each stretch to a point of mild tension for ten seconds, then release. Repeat the stretch three times. Each time you stretch, go a little farther. Go as far as you can as long as you're comfortable and you don't feel any pain.

**Upper Shoulder Towel-Lift Exercise**

You can prevent shoulder pain and fatigue with this easy exercise.

1. Stand with your legs hip width apart then move one foot forward, with the toes pointing straight ahead. Bend your front knee so that it's directly over your ankle; this will cause your rear leg to straighten. Keep both feet on the floor. You'll feel like you're leaning forward, but try to distribute your body weight equally over both legs. Do *not* lock your knees. You are now in a full-lunge position.

2. Hold each end of your towel in each hand, with your arms straight out in front of you.

3. Pull on the ends of the towel, as if trying to tear it apart, until your arms are at least shoulder width apart. Now lift your arms upward, keeping them straight, until your elbows are slightly behind your ears. If this is uncomfortable, raise your arms as high as you find comfortable. Maintain the tension on the towel as you lower it back to the starting position.

4. Maintain the full-lunge position throughout the exercise.

Do as many repetitions as you feel like without straining the muscles in your arms and legs. This exercise can also be done in a seated position, provided you can balance your weight while seated and nothing (arms on the chair, for example) will interfere with your arm movement.

**Chest Towel-Lift Exercise**

This exercise will gently stretch the muscles in your chest and shoulders, which often become tight, especially at night or in the early morning and especially if you sleep on your side.

1. Start in the same position as the previous exercise, but shift your body weight to the back leg so that your torso is upright and balanced between both legs. Keeping your front knee bent, bend your back knee slightly, keeping both feet flat on the floor.

2. Contract your abdominal muscles and tilt your pelvis forward, so that you feel as if your tailbone were pointing toward the floor.

3. With the palms of your hands facing forward, hold the towel by its ends behind your back. Keep your arms straight, but avoid locking your elbows.

4. Pulling on both ends of the towel as if trying to pull it apart, lift the towel behind you slowly until it is behind your lower back. As

you lift, keep your pelvis tucked under so that you don't arch your lower back.

5.  Lower the towel slowly to the starting position, keeping mild tension on the towel.

Repeat this exercise as many times as you feel comfortable, without putting undo strain on your chest, shoulders, arms, or back. This exercise can also be done in a seated position, provided you can balance your weight properly and nothing (a chair back, for example), will interfere with your arm movement.

***Seated Towel Hamstring-Stretch Exercise***

1.  Sit on the floor with your back against a wall, legs in front of you but slightly bent, and a pillow under your left thigh.

2.  Bend your right leg along the floor, so that the sole of your right foot rests against your left thigh and your right knee rests on the floor (or as close as it can get to the floor).

3.  Place the towel around your left heel and hold both ends in your left hand, keeping your right hand on the floor near your right hip for balance.

4.  Maintain tension on the towel and an erect sitting position as you straighten your left knee, flexing your foot and pressing through the heel.

5.  Repeat several times, then relax.

6.  Switch leg positions, then do the same exercise with the towel around your right leg.

***Towel Calf-Strengthening Exercise***

This exercise will strengthen your calf muscles and prevent swelling in your legs, feet, and ankles.

1.  Sit on the floor with your back against the wall, your right leg extended, and your left leg bent.

2.  Wrap a towel around the ball of your right foot, holding the ends of the towel with both hands. Pull the towel taut, keeping your arms close to your sides.

3.  Maintaining tension on the towel, raise your right leg off the floor about 30 degrees, keeping it extended. Relax, then repeat.

4.  Repeat the exercise using your left leg.

## Yoga

You may have heard about yoga instructors who do headstands an hour before labor and then deliver a perfectly healthy (and smiling) baby in less than ten minutes.

While these stories may be true, we don't recommend headstands for you. Gentle yoga exercises, however, are safe and easy to do. We've incorporated three of them into your daily relaxation/exercise program. We recommend that you begin with five repetitions and gradually work up to twenty. Breathe slowly and rhythmically during each movement, and be careful not to strain any muscles. This is a safe workout for pregnant women, even if you haven't done yoga before.

### *Knee-Chest Exercise*

This exercise not only eases backaches, it also improves circulation and relieves gas and constipation.

1. Start with your hands and knees on the floor, with a large cushion between your hands and underneath your chest.

2. Slowly bend your elbows until they rest on the floor. Let your head rest on the cushion.

3. Your back should feel rounded and comfortable. Move your knees apart and forward a bit, if necessary, to achieve this feeling. Hold this position for five to ten seconds, then relax.

4. To get up, push against your hands, stretching your arms until they are almost straight, then slowly uncurl your spine until you're sitting on your knees.

### *Kneeling Pelvic Tilt Exercise*

This exercise may prevent back pain and improve your posture. You may feel the benefits almost instantly.

1. Start with your hands and knees on the floor with your back relaxed.

2. Inhale slowly, tucking your tailbone under so that your back is completely rounded.

3. Hold for a count of three.

4. Exhale and relax.

5. Repeat a total of five times, gradually increasing the number of repetitions and the hold count each time.

**Shoulder Circles**    Practicing this exercise while standing or sitting may help relieve fatigue, upper back pain, and stiffness in your shoulders.

1. Shrug both shoulders, then release them.
2. Lift both shoulders and circle them toward your back, down, and toward the front.
3. Lift one shoulder and rotate it slowly in a full circular motion.
4. Let the shoulder drop and totally relax.
5. Repeat with the other shoulder.

## Calisthenics Pregnancy Exercise

Even if you can't join an organized exercise program, you can still stay fit by practicing simple calisthenics at home to gently strengthen your lower back and your pelvic, abdominal, and leg muscles. As with the yoga exercises, we recommend that you combine these exercises with the relaxation breathing exercises described in Chapter 5. Take a minute to let your breath return to normal before you stand up or proceed to the next exercise. Always work within your capacity. If you experience any discomfort, stop and do a relaxation exercise.

**Chair Straddle Abdominals Exercise**    This is a safe abdominal exercise that you can do throughout your pregnancy, even during labor.

1. Place a pillow against the back of a straight-back, armless chair, so that its upper edge lies over the top of the chair.
2. Facing the back of the chair, straddle the seat.
3. Sit as far forward as possible, keeping both feet planted firmly on the floor.
4. Contract your abdominal muscles and tuck your tailbone under, thus tilting your pelvis forward.
5. Keeping your back straight, lengthen your torso and bring both arms overhead, using one hand to hold the other wrist.
6. Breathe deeply, then exhale. As you exhale, bend your upper body (head, neck, arms, and shoulders) forward. Bend to the point where you feel a gentle stretch.
7. Rest your chin on the pillow and cross your arms in front of you, as if trying to hug the back of the chair. (If that's uncomfortable, simply lower your arms while continuing to hold your wrist.)
8. Relax and hold the stretch for another thirty seconds.

*Seated Back-Stretching Exercise*

This exercise combines yoga breathing exercises with stretches for the upper and lower back.

1. Place a pillow against the back of an armless chair, so that its upper end lies over the top of the chair.

2. Straddle the chair while facing the back of it. Keep your feet planted on the floor.

3. Bring both arms around the back of the chair, and interlock your fingers.

4. Lean forward and place your forehead on the pillow.

5. Push down into your heels, contracting your buttocks and rounding your spine.

*Kneeling Abdominals Exercise*

This exercise gently stretches your neck and middle and lower back muscles, and is designed to help keep your spine aligned.

1. Kneel on a pillow placed in front of a low bed or chair.

2. Sit on your heels with your feet close together and your knees far enough apart to accommodate your belly.

3. Cross your arms in front of you, and lean your upper body forward so that your head touches the edge of the bed or chair. Your head should be down, either with your crown facing forward or your head turned to the side.

4. If you tend to get leg or foot cramps, put another pillow behind your knees and don't sit too far back on your heels. Also, try turning your feet out if that's more comfortable.

*Lower-Back/Leg Stretches*

This exercise stretches your lower back and hamstring muscles, and is designed to relieve sciatica and lower-back pain.

1. Lie on your left side on the floor or in bed.

2. Place a pillow under your head and one or two pillows between your legs. Keep your left arm comfortably in front of you and lower than your shoulder. Don't lie directly on your arm, as this may cause it to go to sleep.

3. Bend both knees and bring them toward your chest. Place your right arm over your right leg, and grasp the back of your right thigh.

4. Pull your right leg closer to your body, and hold for a count of ten.

5. As you bring your leg towards you, you should feel your lower back rounding. Gently contract your abdominal muscles while relaxing your hips. Do three or four repetitions.

6. Roll over to your right side and repeat this exercise with the other leg. Finish by taking a deep breath and relaxing for thirty seconds.

*Back/Calf/ Hamstring Stretch*

You need to exercise your legs continually throughout pregnancy to prevent varicose veins. Try this exercise every day.

1. Sit with your left leg bent and your right leg stretched out in front of you.

2. With your arms stretched out in front of you, slowly reach forward over your right leg from your hips and stretch your right calf and hamstring muscles as much as your belly will permit.

3. Repeat the exercise, with your left leg.

*Demi Plié*

This exercise is designed to tone the back of your thighs and your knee ligaments.

1. Stand with your feet about two feet apart, your toes turned comfortably out. Place one hand on a chair back, hand rail, or wall for support.

2. Slowly bend your knees, keeping your back straight. Keep your knees over your toes; don't let them roll in.

3. Rise slowly, concentrating on the calf muscles as you push upward. Your heels should remain on the floor throughout the entire movement.

4. Keep rising until your legs are straight again. If you feel that you have a keen sense of balance, continue rising until you are on the balls of your feet. Then slowly descend until your feet are flat on the floor again.

## Weight-Lifting Exercises

Light weight lifting, using dumbbells weighing no more than five pounds, may be very helpful for preventing pain in your shoulders, upper and lower back, arms, and thighs during pregnancy. In place of dumbbells, you can use water bottles or sugar bags. Make sure that you don't hold your breath while lifting weights, since this diminishes blood flow to your baby.

**Shoulder Raises**

Your growing abdomen can make you stoop forward, causing shoulder pain. This exercise may help strengthen muscles in your shoulders and arms.

1. Sit in a straight-back chair. Hold a dumbbell in each hand with your palms facing your body and your arms down at your sides. Keep your elbows slightly bent and wrists locked.

2. Lean forward from the hips, letting your arms hang until they are next to your thighs.

3. Squeeze your shoulder blades together to bring your arms outward to shoulder height.

4. Lower your arms to the starting position and repeat. Try to keep your torso motionless as you lift your arms.

**Mid-Back–Stretching Exercise**

This exercise is designed to strengthen your mid-back and rear shoulder muscles.

1. Sit in a straight-back chair with your feet hip width apart and your left foot twelve inches in front of your right.

2. Hold a dumbbell in your right hand with your wrist locked and palm facing inward. Try to keep your arm straight and hanging down directly in line with your shoulder.

3. While squeezing your shoulder blades down and together, lift your right arm up and out until your elbow is in line with your shoulder.

4. Slowly return your arm to the starting position, and repeat.

5. Relax, then repeat this exercise using the other arm.

## Holistic Approaches to Common Third-Month Concerns

Holistic pregnancy is all about feeling happy and healthy in mind and body. That doesn't mean you won't get a headache or neck pain every now and then. Here are a few holistic methods that may help keep them to a minimum.

## HOLISTIC EXERCISE PROGRAM

We recommend that you do three exercises a day—fifteen minutes per exercise, including repetitions. You'll find that they get easier and easier and that you'll be able to gradually increase the duration of each exercise (if you have available time). Here's a suggested weekly workout schedule.

**Monday**

Standing Kegel Exercise

Upper Shoulder Towel-Lift Exercise

Knee-Chest Exercise

**Tuesday**

Lying-Down Kegel Exercise

Chest Towel-Lift Exercise

Kneeling Pelvic Tilt Exercise

**Wednesday**

Shoulder Circles

Towel Calf-Strengthening Exercise

Chair Straddle Abdominals Exercise

**Thursday**

Seated Back-Stretching Exercise

Mid-Back–Stretching Exercise

Shoulder Raises

**Friday**

Kneeling Abdominals Exercise

Demi Plié

Back/Calf/Hamstring Stretch

**Saturday**

Seated Towel Hamstring-Stretch Exercise

Lower-Back/Leg Stretches

## Tension Headaches

Headaches may result from the physical or psychological stresses of pregnancy. Tension headaches are caused by sustained constriction of scalp, neck, and facial muscles and are marked by tightness and pressure in the forehead and the back of the head and neck.

Poor posture often causes tension headaches by reducing the spaces between the vertebrae (bones of the spine in the neck), putting the squeeze on blood vessels that pass through them. Exercises designed to correct and maintain proper posture will, in turn, help maintain adequate separation between the vertebrae.

Tension headaches can be triggered by strained neck muscles. Learning to keep your head upright without overstressing your neck muscles may help prevent neck pain and neck-related headaches.

For tension headaches caused by poor posture, midwives advise women to practice balancing a folded towel on the top of their heads. This will teach you to keep your head and neck properly aligned, and help relax your shoulders. Try the towel trick for a few minutes each day as you go about your normal routine.

**Acupressure**
You also can relieve tension and migraine headaches by gently pressing acupressure points in the eye socket (with your eye closed). You can do this by locating the halfway point between the outer corner of the eye and outer end of your eyebrow. Your finger should be on a ridge of bone, which is the outer edge of your eye socket. Move one finger's width back toward the center of your nose and gently massage, applying gentle, stroking pressure.

**Biofeedback**
Minor tension headaches can also be relieved with biofeedback. One simple method you can use at home is to sit quietly, close your eyes, and visualize raising the temperature of your fingers or hands. This helps draw blood from your head, allowing blood vessels to shrink and thereby easing headaches.

**Aromatherapy**
Massaging the spine, shoulders, neck, and head with lavender and almond oil may relieve most types of headache. You can also add a few drops of lavender oil to your evening bath.

**Osteopathy**
Cranial sacral osteopathy is a simple and safe way of relieving tension headaches due to tension in spinal muscles. Be sure to consult an osteopath who specializes in treating pregnant women.

**Deep Breathing**
The diaphragmatic breathing exercises discussed in Chapter 3 serve as another way to prevent tension headaches. Deep-breathing exercises help release endorphins, which relieve pain. If you practice your breathing exercises routinely, you may have fewer headaches.

**Hot Showers**
Midwives have found that taking a quick hot shower followed immediately by a brief cold shower helps relieve headaches for some women. The drops of water trigger the release of endorphins throughout the body to stimulate relaxation.

## Migraine Headaches

Nothing sabotages your mind/body health faster than a migraine headache. Migraines are intense, one-sided, throbbing headaches that can make you nauseous. They're usually preceded by *auras,* or visual changes (such as double vision or a halo of light around objects). Symptoms vary, but usually include fatigue followed by nausea, with or without vomiting, and diarrhea. Some women also experience tingling or numbness in one arm or one side of the body, as well as dizziness, ringing in the ears, a runny nose, or bloodshot eyes.

Migraines can be extremely painful. An accurate diagnosis of the causes of migraines is essential for effective treatment, so if they persist, work with your caregiver to identify the causes. The following remedies have been used to prevent or relieve migraines. You may find some of them helpful.

### Bach Flower Remedies

A combination of gentian, water violet, walnut, and Bach's emergency stress remedies has been used to relieve migraine headaches. These can be taken as tinctures or inhaled through an infusion. They should be prescribed by a Bach therapist or your caregiver.

### Botanical Medicine

Canadian midwives have given feverfew capsules and teas to prevent and reverse migraine attacks.

### Deep Breathing

The following breathing exercise may relieve tension and, as a result, migraines.

1. Close your eyes, center yourself, and breathe from the abdomen.

2. Imagine your inhaled breath as loving attention, and breathe through the pain.

3. As you breathe out, imagine you are pushing the pain out of your head.

### Physical Activity

Running and other forms of aerobic activity are effective ways for some people to relieve migraine headaches, because it increases the production of endorphins.

### Massage

The following simple method of self-massage may also relieve migraine headaches.

1. Place the fingers of both hands on either side of the midline along the back of your neck, just under your skull.

2. Keeping your fingers perpendicular to the neck midline and your elbows up, apply pressure to your neck muscles with your fingertips.

3. Stroke the neck upward and apply pressure deep into the neck muscles.

4. Exhale, and let your head fall back into your fingers as your elbows descend, pulling your hands forward. Massage individual muscle fibers with your fingers as your hands glide forward. You may also find massaging down the neck muscles helpful. Massaging across the muscles, the standard shiatsu technique, is more effective for removing energy blockages, however.

## "Digestive" Headaches

Some headaches are referred to as *digestive headaches,* because they are caused by food sensitivities or by not eating at least three regular meals a day. Digestive headaches usually settle in right behind the eyes. The following massage may help ease the symptoms:

1. Use your left hand to find the sensitive spot in the webbing between your thumb and index finger of your right hand.

2. Press this spot with your thumb and forefinger—this should produce a sharp twinge.

3. If the headache lingers, repeat the procedure one or two more times by pressing the webbing of your left hand.

### Brush Massage

Poor cranial circulation often causes headaches. Stimulating the scalp with a hair or bath brush can relieve symptoms by increasing circulation in the skin. The entire surface of the scalp should be brushed gently, with downward strokes from the top of the head.

### Nutrition and Supplements

Digestive headaches also can be relieved by avoiding salty and acid-producing foods. If you suffer frequent headaches, consult a nutritionist for a *rotation diet* to eliminate irritating foods. Some women may benefit from eliminating milk and milk products, or yellow cheese specifically, and cherries. Nitrates, which are used as preservatives in hot dogs and luncheon meats, should also be avoided. Aged cheese, wine, beer, chocolate, vinegar, pickles, organ meats, preserved fish and meat, soy and lima beans, onions, spinach, and foods with MSG (monosodium glutamate) should also be eliminated to see if they are the cause of headache. Good foods to consume are yogurt (if you're not allergic to milk or milk products) and cereals.

## Neck Pains

It's hard enough learning how to find a comfortable position for sleeping during pregnancy without having to suffer neck pain. This type of pain is usually caused by muscle tension. Your chiropractor or osteopath may easily relieve it.

To relieve neck pain on your own, try this quickie stretch exercise at home or at work. You can do it at your desk, in a taxi—even in bed before you go to sleep.

1. Sit or stand with your back, head, and neck in as straight a line as possible.

2. Slowly tilt your head forward, trying to touch your chin to your chest.

3. Lift one bent arm so that your elbow is pointing skyward and your palm is resting on the base of your skull.

4. Use the other arm to gently pull your head down, exhaling as you feel the stretch. Hold the stretch for several seconds, inhale, and repeat two to four times.

To stretch the sides of your neck,

1. Slowly tilt your head sideways, attempting to touch your right ear to your right shoulder without raising your shoulder.

2. Raise your right arm over your head, placing your palm on your left ear, and gently pull your head toward your shoulders.

3. Hold the stretch for two seconds, and repeat two to four times on each side.

The combination of the movement, stretching, and breathing should relieve tension right away.

### Acupressure

Acupressure can relieve neck pain due to many causes, especially constriction of blood vessels to the head. It will also relax stiff shoulders and prevent the headaches often associated with neck pain.

### Neck Exercise

You can use this exercise to gently relax your neck and shoulders.

1. Sit in a comfortable position with your eyes closed and your head dropped forward.

2. Inhale slowly using yoga breathing, and gently roll your head to the right until your ear is above your right shoulder.

3. Exhale and relax, letting your head drop forward comfortably again.

4. Repeat four or five times, alternating the direction of the roll and relaxing between rolls.

The best way to guarantee that you stay fit throughout pregnancy is to join an exercise class. If you can't, you can still keep in shape by following our simple home Holistic Exercise Program. It's convenient, inexpensive, stimulating, and great for your muscles and cardiovascular system. You can do it in the fresh air, alone, or with friends. And you don't have to worry about gym membership fees, teammates who can cancel at the last minute, or having to get there. So there's no reason not to try to keep in shape and give your baby the best chance for being born healthy!

## Chapter 5

# The Fourth Month

*W*ELCOME TO YOUR SECOND TRIMESTER!

By the fourth month of pregnancy, your baby weighs about three ounces and is approximately four inches long. Your abdomen is expanding noticeably, and you'll soon be looking for looser clothing to wear. You may already have felt your baby's movements, called *quickening*.

Your baby is swallowing and excreting amniotic fluid, which surrounds the baby and cushions him or her to prevent injury. By the sixteenth week, fecal matter, called *meconium,* will begin collecting in the baby's intestinal tract.

## *T*HE FOURTH-MONTH CHECKUP

During your fourth-month checkup, your caregiver will continue to monitor your baby's heartbeat as well as your weight, blood pressure, and urine, along with the size of your uterus and the height of your fundus, while checking for signs of edema (swelling) and varicose veins. This is usually a comfortable month for most women. Nevertheless, you may develop the occasional headache, nose bleed, indigestion, or hemorrhoids. Be sure to mention these to your caregiver and discuss holistic remedies for them.

This chapter stresses the importance of avoiding potential toxins and outlines a safe and effective detoxification program designed to protect both you and your baby.

## MINIMIZING YOUR EXPOSURE TO HARMFUL TOXINS

There has never been a time in history when having a baby was safer. Obstetricians are now better equipped than ever before to deal with high-risk pregnancies and keep alive babies born as much as two months premature.

You know, however, that living in a modern society means that you're more likely than ever before to be exposed to harmful toxins—while driving to and from work, inside the office or factory, eating or shopping, or even carrying out simple household chores. Just as you wouldn't think of becoming pregnant downstream from a nuclear reactor, holistic practitioners are adamant about your avoiding all toxins. Toxins are found everywhere, including the air you breathe, the water you drink, and the food you eat. We recommend that you minimize your exposure to any unsafe substances—both for your sake and the sake of your baby. We don't want you to *worry;* we want you to feel *safe.* You'll eliminate many hours of worrying later (and potential birth defects) if you take the time now to follow the precautions outlined below.

### Air Pollution

The air in many industrialized countries is now severely polluted. The ability of smog to produce birth defects has not yet been proven, but it can't hurt to play it safe. If you live in a very smoggy area, use an air purifier and don't go outside during smog alerts.

### Lead Poisoning

Studies have also documented that women who work with lead in factories suffer higher rates of sterility, miscarriage, and premature births, and are more likely than others to have babies born with birth defects. If your home was built in 1955 or earlier, it may have been painted with lead-based paint. If so, consider having the paint replaced. Until then, stay away from the house when any construction is being done or any old paint is removed. Also, avoid your partner if he works with old paint until he has showered and replaced his work clothes. Ask your local environmental safety office to test the lead levels in your drinking water, and avoid serving food or drink in earthenware, pottery, or china contaminated by lead. That means avoiding pitchers or dishes that are home crafted, imported, antique, or that contain lead crystal.

## Immunotoxins

Some immunotoxic chemicals—such as industrial gases, asbestos, and silica—readily find their way into the human bloodstream and weaken the immune system. Your body cannot eliminate these immunotoxic pollutants; therefore, you should avoid them whenever possible. For example, avoid any task that exposes you to gas fumes or asbestos or silicon products.

## Extremely-Low-Frequency (ELF) Electromagnetic Fields

Recent studies in Sweden have shown that direct exposure during pregnancy to electromagnetic fields (EMFs) generated by high-voltage power lines can cause leukemia in children. Don't take a chance: contact the EPA or your local city government and find out what the voltage and dangers are. If you live next to a high-voltage power line, move to another location, if possible, at least until your baby is born.

Older electrically heated waterbeds have been linked to miscarriages due to EMFs. Use a newer, super-low EMF waterbed heater. If you have an older heater, warm the bed ahead of time, then turn the heater off before you get into bed.

## X Rays

Diagnostic x rays are dangerous for your baby. If possible, postpone unnecessary x rays or computed tomographic (CT) scans until after delivery. If an x ray is necessary, always tell the doctor or radiology technician that you're pregnant, and make sure you are properly shielded with a lead apron.

## Radioactive Gases

Exposure to high concentrations of radioactive gases can cause cancer. The most common dangerous radioactive gas in the United States is radon, a naturally occurring gas released from certain rocks (especially granite) and building materials, such as concrete, bricks, and tiles. The Environmental Protection Agency (EPA) now advises expectant mothers to contact their local authorities or ecological groups to determine if they live in a radon-contaminated area. Since approximately 6 percent of American homes have elevated radon levels, you may want to buy a radon detector to monitor radon levels in yours.

## Drinking Water

More than 100 potentially toxic chemicals have been identified in local water supplies in the United States. Several are carcinogenic (cancer causing), including benzene, carbon tetrachloride, dioxin, ethylene dibromide (EDB), polychlorinated biphenyls (PCBs), and vinyl chloride. These and other toxins may be introduced into your town's water supply through contamination with waste, pesticides, or specific toxins, or by the leaching of metals from copper or lead pipes. Toxic levels of heavy metals can result in mental retardation in children and nervous system disorders in adults and children. As a precaution, check with your local EPA or health department about the purity and safety of your community water supply. Have your water tested by the local EPA or health department. If it is not safe, use bottled water for all drinking and cooking. If you must use tap water, use only cold water for drinking and cooking (hot water leaches more lead from the pipes). If the water has not been turned on for six hours or more, run the cold-water tap for five minutes before using it. Boiling your tap water or letting it stand for twenty-four hours helps to evaporate harmful chemicals, such as lead. Otherwise, install an FDA-approved water filter and drink only filtered water.

## Food Toxins

Some of the foods you purchase at the local grocery store may contain toxins; these include fruits and vegetables treated with pesticides, insecticides, larvicides, or herbicides. Meats from animals raised on hormones *may* cause infertility, impotence, neurological disorders, cancer, and birth defects. The safest bet is to eat only fresh, organically grown foods, which are available from health food stores and some supermarkets.

## Microbial Toxins

The bacteria that normally live in the intestines produce toxic substances to protect themselves. These substances include endotoxins and exotoxins. In addition, toxic amines from protein metabolism and toxic derivatives of bile can accumulate in blood and other tissues. These toxins can prevent the development of antibodies, which normally fight infections. These toxins rarely reach harmful levels in

## PREVENTING FOOD CONTAMINATION

1. Remove the outer leaves of leafy vegetables and peel the waxy coating off fruits and vegetables.

2. Wash all hard-skinned produce in very diluted dishwashing liquid, then rinse well.

3. Eat yogurt with live bacillus to reduce your vulnerability to harmful organisms. Yogurt contains bacteria that help maintain healthy intestinal flora and limit the growth of harmful organisms, including other bacteria such as *Salmonella* and *Listeria*.

4. Avoid out-of-season fruits and vegetables, which may carry twice the risk of pesticide and fungicide contamination. Ninety percent of fungicides are carcinogenic.

5. When washing your hands before handling food, be sure to clean under your fingernails.

6. Vegetable oils can become rancid with exposure to air, heat, or light. Oils should be stored in small, dark bottles rather than in partially empty large bottles to reduce their exposure to oxygen.

pregnant mothers. As a precaution, however, ask your caregiver to periodically test your blood for them.

## Toxins in the Workplace

Inside a typical office building there are likely to be at least 50 (possibly as many as 500) volatile organic compounds (VOCs) and gases, which are emitted by everything from caulking to carpeting. According to the EPA, most office pollution results from harmful gases released from materials used in newly constructed or recently renovated buildings. Many gases cannot be detected by odor. Some indoor air pollutants cause asthma, hypersensitivity pneumonitis, and *multiple chemical sensitivity* disorders, all of which can destroy the immune system. Common symptoms include dizziness, headaches, nausea, burning eyes, nosebleeds, fatigue, excessive coughing and sneezing, and itchy skin and throat.

## Toxins in Your Home

Your home may also contain toxins—even from relatively innocent sources. Ordinary building materials used in walls, floors, insulation, roofs, paint, plastic tiles, and carpets are often toxic and can cause flulike symptoms, such as weakness, aching joints, congestion, nosebleeds, and dizziness. Ask the local EPA office to recommend a consultant to inspect your home for toxins, and replace toxic materials with nontoxic substitutes, where possible.

Although there's no evidence that the typical levels of toxins in your home are harmful to either you or your baby, you'll be more comfortable in the long run knowing that you've done everything you can to prepare a safe and natural environment for your baby. Don't paint or even wallpaper baby's room when you're pregnant, because this may release toxic gases. And be sure to air out any new carpet or rugs months before baby is due. And try the *green solution*—filling your home with house plants. Plants absorb carbon dioxide in the air while adding oxygen and, of course, beauty, to your indoor environment.

## Microwave Ovens

Leaking microwave ovens that dissipate heat can potentially harm your fetus. Make sure your oven doesn't leak, and don't operate it if the seals around the door are damaged, the door doesn't close properly, or if something is caught in the door. You can also ask an appliance service center, your city or state consumer protection office, or your local health department to test your oven for safety. And don't stand in front of the oven when it's operating.

## Electric Blankets and Heating Pads

There is no conclusive evidence that electric blankets or heating pads can harm your fetus. However, as a precaution, wrap heating pads in a towel to reduce heat, limit applications to fifteen minutes, and don't sleep with them. It's safer to use alternative sources of warmth, such as flannel sheets, heaters, and dressing in layers.

# HOLISTIC APPROACHES TO STRENGTHENING THE IMMUNE SYSTEM

Realistically, it may not be possible for you to protect yourself against *all* potential toxins, especially environmental toxins such as smog or carbon dioxide. Their overall effect on your pregnancy will be less if you focus on factors that you can control, such as exercising regularly, adopting a holistic food plan, and avoiding alcohol, smoking, and recreational drugs.

## HOLISTIC PREGNANCY PROGRAM: ELIMINATING TOXINS IN YOUR HOME

### In the Kitchen:

Check product labels and don't use

▷ Paper towels fortified with formaldehyde, which can cause skin rashes, nausea, and eye and lung irritation

▷ Bleached paper containing dioxin

▷ Air fresheners containing carbolic acid or formaldehyde, which can cause nausea

▷ Oven cleaners containing lye, phenols, formaldehyde, benzene, or ammonia, which can cause blisters and rashes

### In Bathrooms

Check labels and don't use

▷ Antiperspirants containing aluminum chlorohydrate, which blocks skin pores

▷ Commercial toothpastes that contain ammonia, ethanol, formaldehyde, mineral oil, or saccharin

▷ Furniture and tile polish containing sodium phosphate or turpentine, which can burn the skin and is dangerous when inhaled

▷ Toilet cleaners containing cresol, which is easily absorbed through the skin and can damage major organs

### For Clothing

Check labels and don't use

▷ Leather shoe dyes containing nitrobenzene, which can turn the skin blue, affects breathing, and induces vomiting

▷ Spot removers containing benzene, sulfuric acid, or toluene, which can cause skin rashes and nervous system complications.

Ask your dry cleaner if he uses benzene, sulfuric acid, or toluene. Dry-cleaned clothes not exposed to these are safe.

### At the Office

Don't use

▷ Polyester padded partitions, curtains, or carpets

▷ Photocopying machines that give off ozone

▷ Blueprint copiers that give off ammonia and acetic acid vapors, causing eye, nose, and throat irritation

### Recommendations

Do use

▷ Natural, nontoxic products, such as corn starch or arrowroot instead of talc

▷ Bicarbonate of soda, peppermint oil, or natural herb toothpastes

▷ Essential oil deodorants instead of strong chemical deodorants

▷ Natural, nontoxic antidandruff shampoos

▷ For housecleaning, use a mixture of ten drops of citrus/ylang oil in two quarts of tap water to kill airborne bacteria and leave your rooms with a fresh, delightful aroma; baking soda mixed with water to scrub tubs and tiles.

▷ While traveling, use essential oils and fragrances to stay alert and prevent motion sickness: Spray the car's interior with them to stay focused and alert, to take advantage of their antiseptic qualities (which make them useful in restrooms and hotels), or to feel refreshed after a nap.

Our holistic program emphasizes strengthening your immune system with vitamin, mineral, and herbal supplements that have been proven effective in detoxification. Vitamin $B_6$ and vitamin K, glutamate, magnesium citrate, and potassium citrate have been used to help detoxify the kidneys. Cranberry juice has been used to control bacterial growth along the urinary tract. Aloe vera juice and *lactobacillus acidophillus* (the bacteria found in natural yogurt) may help preserve the natural microflora (bacteria) in your intestines. Small amounts of fresh garlic, cider vinegar, and barberry plant supplements may help prevent intestinal infections.

Herbs that help eliminate toxins from your colon include alfalfa, bentonite, goldenseal, echinacea, buckthorn, cassia senna leaves, and psyllium seed powder mixed with water. Goldenseal, echinacea, ginseng, or licorice may help improve lymphatic drainage. Discuss the role of these nutrients in your daily food plan with your caregiver, nutritionist, or herbalist.

## Nutrition and Supplements

Ask your caregiver if you should take any of the following supplements to enhance your immune system: vitamins A, B complex, C, E, zinc, copper, selenium, acidophilus/megadophilus, coenzyme $Q_{10}$, garlic capsules, germanium, or spirulina.

# HOLISTIC BREATHING AND RELAXATION EXERCISES

Your mind/body health depends on reversing the stress response—by inducing the relaxation response. This section provides simple instructions for several relaxation exercises: abdominal breathing, affirmations, meditation, progressive relaxation, white-light visualization, receptive imagery, and programmed imagery. These exercises trigger the *relaxation response;* that is, they stimulate the release of endorphins, the body's natural tranquilizers, which can be as powerful (or even more so) as prescription drugs, without the side effects. When practiced every day, these exercises may help relieve the pain and discomfort you may experience during pregnancy, labor, and childbirth. According to Dr. Howard Shapiro in his book, *The Pregnancy Book for Today's Woman,* they also stimulate your baby's growth and development.

## FOODS THAT ENHANCE YOUR IMMUNE SYSTEM

During the last twenty years, numerous studies have documented that certain vitamin- and mineral-rich foods help strengthen your immune system.

▷ **Foods rich in vitamins A and C.** Vitamin C is essential for several immune functions, including normal white blood cell activity, interferon levels, and increasing antibody levels and response. Vitamin A helps the body resist respiratory infections and is important for maintaining healthy skin, hair, and mucous membranes. The best food sources of vitamins A and C are dark green leafy vegetables, broccoli, and citrus fruits.

▷ **Foods rich in beta carotene.** Beta carotene, a substance from which the body makes vitamin A, triggers the antitumor activity of *macrophages,* the white blood cells that engulf and destroy bacteria and other invaders. Excellent food sources include deep yellow, orange, or green vegetables and fruits, such as beets, mustard greens, turnip greens, carrots, chili peppers, pumpkins, spinach, winter squash, apricots, cantaloupes, mangoes, papayas, and peaches.

▷ **Foods rich in vitamin E.** Vitamin E helps increase the production of *interleukin-2,* a naturally occurring substance that works mainly in the lymphatic system to bolster immune function. Nuts, sunflower seeds, wheat germ, and vegetable oils are excellent sources.

▷ **Foods rich in zinc.** Zinc is the best-known activator of the thymus gland, which helps produce T cells. Seafood, especially oysters, is an excellent source of zinc.

▷ **Foods rich in iron, selenium, folate, and vitamin $B_6$.** A deficiency of vitamin $B_6$ depresses all immune functions, and an iron deficiency increases susceptibility to infection. Selenium and folate boost immune function. Animal meats and fish are natural sources of iron; dried beans and iron-enriched cereals are excellent non-meat sources. Bananas, cantaloupe, lemons, oranges, and strawberries are good fruit sources of folate; good vegetable sources include asparagus, broccoli, lima beans, and spinach. The best sources of selenium are high-protein foods, such as meats, as well as cereal and milk and milk products. White meats, such as chicken and fish, are the richest sources of vitamin $B_6$, as are whole grains and potatoes.

*Adapted from* Joseph Pizzorno and Michael Murray, *Encyclopedia of Natural Medicine;* and James Marti, *Alternative Health and Medicine Encyclopedia.*

To help you get started, we've integrated thirteen exercises into a Weekly Holistic Relaxation Program recommended by our Medical Advisory Board. By efficiently managing your time, you should be able to follow the Program without any difficulty. At the outset, try to follow the recommended time period for each exercise. Once you're familiar with each exercise, you can shorten the time period to fit your daily schedule and select the exercises you respond to best. To help you stick with these throughout your whole pregnancy, we've divided the Program into alternate days to keep you from getting bored. You can practice many of these simple exercises at the office, or while riding a bus, standing in line at the grocery store, or cleaning house.

The sequence of relaxation exercises will help stimulate your internal healing powers. They are always, as Albert Schweitzer once suggested, "activating the doctor within."

---

## HOLISTIC PREGNANCY RELAXATION PROGRAM

### Monday, Wednesday, and Friday

**Morning**
Abdominal breathing with affirmations:
    5 minutes
Zen breathing: 3–5 minutes
Meditation: 3–5 minutes
Sound, touch, or color meditation:
    3 minutes

**Afternoon**
(At least one hour after lunch)
Abdominal breathing with affirmations:
    5 minutes
Sound, touch, or color meditation:
    3 minutes
White-light visualization: 3 minutes
Receptive imagery: 3 minutes

**Evening**
(At least one hour after dinner)
Abdominal breathing with affirmations:
    5 minutes
Counting meditation: 3 minutes
Alternate-nostril breathing: 3 minutes
Relaxation massage: 5 minutes

### Tuesday, Thursday, Saturday, and Sunday

**Morning**
Abdominal breathing with affirmations:
    5 minutes
Zen breathing: 3 minutes
Simple meditation: 3 minutes
Sound, touch, or color meditation: 3 minutes

**Afternoon**
(At least one hour after lunch)
Abdominal breathing with affirmations:
    5 minutes
Sound, touch, or color meditation:
    3 minutes
Progressive relaxation: 3 minutes
Programmed imagery: 3 minutes

**Evening**
(At least one hour after dinner)
Abdominal breathing with affirmations:
    5 minutes
Sound, touch, or color meditation: 3 minutes
Alternate-nostril breathing: 3 minutes

## Abdominal Breathing

You cannot function at your best during pregnancy and labor if you do not breathe correctly. In his book, *Childbirth Without Fear,* Grantly Dick-Read suggests that incorrect breathing actually causes more complications during labor and childbirth than anything else. The key to correct breathing, according to Dick-Read, is controlling how you breathe in fresh air and exhale stale waste gases. When you breathe in slowly, more fresh air enters your lungs and more enters your blood for transport to the brain and other organs. The more oxygen that reaches your brain, especially the frontal lobes, the more relaxed you'll be.

Most pregnant women tend to breathe from the upper chest because their abdomens are enlarged. Chest-breathers typically use only one third of the available air space in their lungs. To maintain an adequate supply of oxygen, they have to breathe three times faster than women who breathe correctly. Breathing faster means more work for the respiratory muscles and more work for the heart to pump blood throughout the body. During pregnancy, this can become a strain and uncomfortable. Because your oxygen intake depends on correct breathing techniques, you should practice deep, abdominal breathing. Abdominal breathing is also a fast way to eliminate frustration, anger, tension, and fear. It triggers the relaxation response which, in turn, lowers your heart rate and blood pressure. This is an essential holistic feedback cycle that works continually to the advantage of you and your baby.

## Abdominal Breathing Exercise

The following abdominal breathing exercise is taught in many childbirth classes. This type of breathing does two things: it increases blood circulation to the baby in your womb and helps you relax. By practicing this exercise, you'll learn to tell the difference between abdominal breathing and chest breathing so that you can breathe more efficiently, both for you and your baby.

1.  Sit in a straight-back chair. Slide forward a few inches so that you're reclining slightly. Put a pillow behind your lower back for support.

2.  Place one hand palm down on your lower abdomen below your navel and place the other hand on top of it.

3.  Without trying to change your breathing in any way, simply notice whether your belly is expanding or flattening when you inhale. If your belly expands as you breathe in, you're breathing at least partly from the diaphragm. If your belly doesn't move or if it flattens as you inhale, you're breathing too much from your chest.

4.  Take a deep breath in, then blow it out completely through your mouth, like an audible sigh of relief. As you do this, notice how your belly flattens as you squeeze out every last bit of air.

The key to shifting from chest to diaphragmatic breathing is to exhale completely in one breath. That's why we recommend that you exhale *through your mouth* to fully evacuate the lungs. This full exhalation pushes out all the "stale" air from the bottom of the lungs, and the resulting vacuum automatically causes the diaphragm to contract, allowing the abdomen to flatten and forcing most of the air out of the lungs. You'll notice that you need to breathe out deeply only once or twice. Think of it as a sigh of relief. Sighing and yawning both result in a deep air exchange and are the body's ways of letting go of tension and helping eliminate excess carbon dioxide.

You'll find that two or three minutes of abdominal breathing may automatically reduce any fears and negative thoughts. Whenever you become anxious and tense, remember to shift immediately to abdominal breathing. Once you've mastered this, you can do it anywhere, any time—standing in your kitchen, waiting in line, riding an elevator, driving down the highway. After all, you can always breathe.

## Zen Breathing Exercise

Zen breathing is an abdominal breathing exercise that is taught in pregnancy classes in Asia. By consciously practicing this rhythmic breathing exercise throughout the day, you'll turn anxiety into tranquillity.

1.  Find a quiet, comfortable place to sit where you will not be disturbed.

2.  Breathe in slowly through your nose, and breathe out slowly through your mouth.

3. With each breath, concentrate on the feelings, sensations, and changes you experience through breathing. Listen to your breath. Listen to the life-giving sounds of breathing in and breathing out. This will help you tune out other sounds and forget distracting thoughts.

4. After about three minutes, take one last deep breath and end the session. You should feel completely relaxed and refreshed. As you become more proficient with this technique, you will need progressively less time to become relaxed, because your nervous system will have learned a conditioned relaxation response. Just two or three breaths will bring you the benefits of a longer period of meditation. This is why we suggest only three minutes of Zen breathing.

## Alternate-Nostril Breathing Exercise

Yogis and holy men in India spend many years of their lives studying how to breathe correctly, because breathing is considered the foundation from which higher spiritual states are attained. One yogic breathing exercise, called *Nodi Sadhana,* focuses on inhaling and exhaling through alternate nostrils. This slow, meditative breathing technique works like acupuncture—that is, it purifies the *nadis* (channels) along which the prana "flows." In *Quantum Healing,* Dr. Deepak Chopra suggests that this technique helps the brain produce its own natural painkillers, endorphins.

The following alternate-nostril breathing exercise is taught in the Marin County Hospital's Pregnancy Clinic classes in California. It's an excellent exercise to practice when you first wake up in the morning and just before you go to sleep at night.

1. Sit upright on a cushion or a firm chair with your head, neck, and body aligned.

2. Breathe in a relaxed fashion from your diaphragm for three complete breaths. Inhalation and exhalation should be of equal length and should be slow, controlled, and free from sounds or jerks.

3. Inhale again. Close your right nostril with the thumb of your right hand and exhale completely through your left nostril.

4. At the end of the exhalation, close your left nostril with your right index finger and inhale through the right nostril.

5. Repeat this cycle of exhalation with the left nostril and inhalation with the right nostril two more times, always making sure to maintain an equal inhalation and exhalation.

## Meditation

An excellent way to combine abdominal breathing with affirmations is meditation. *Meditation* is a state of focused concentration that produces a heightened sense of inner peace and awareness. There are several forms of meditation, all of which aid in transforming the *stress response* into the *relaxation response*. One way meditating does this is by stimulating the production of alpha and theta waves in the frontal lobes of the brain. This, in turn, helps lower your heart rate and respiration rate as well as your blood pressure. Meditation also helps alleviate abdominal pain, backaches, and insomnia, which often occur during the last trimester of pregnancy.

Meditation is an ideal way for you to set aside time each day to be silent and just relax. If you meditate at least once a day, you'll find you have greater mental composure, an enhanced ability to concentrate, and more energy. Many pregnant women also find that meditating gives them a heightened spiritual awareness.

We suggest you start each day with a short (three-minute) meditation of your choice after doing the breathing exercise. The following is a simple meditation exercise you can do whenever you feel tired or stressed by the physiological and emotional demands of pregnancy.

1. Assume a comfortable position lying on your back or sitting. If you're sitting, keep your spine straight and let your shoulders drop.

2. Close your eyes if it makes you feel more comfortable.

3. Bring your attention to your belly. Let it expand gently on the in-breath and recede on the out-breath.

4. Keep the focus on your breathing, being *with* each in-breath.

5. Every time you breathe out, repeat to yourself:
   *I am calm and relaxed.*
   *The baby feels my calmness and shares it.*

If you practice this exercise every time you wake up, you'll notice that you feel much more peaceful and confident throughout the day. With repetition, your affirmations become automatic. You'll find that your meditations are a kind of mental martial art that protects you and your baby from the stress response. You learn to take a different approach to the events of the day, with the result of feeling more relaxed, confident, and in control of your pregnancy.

## Counting Meditation

In this exercise, you either sit or lie down comfortably in a quiet place. You begin by using either abdominal or alternate-nostril breathing. As you exhale, count out a number, starting at twenty and going backwards (one number with each breath) to help you relax. When you reach "one," silently focus on a key phrase, such as "calm and confident." Repeat your key word or phrase several times with successive breaths. After a while your subconscious mind begins to associate the process with your key words, and you become receptive to these feelings whenever you repeat the exercise.

## Affirmations

As you prepare for your baby's birth, you may have special concerns and fears: the fear, for example, that you'll miscarry or that complications will occur. Fear can be very helpful if it encourages you to take the best possible care of yourself and your baby. The Receptive Imagery section below discusses how you can convert fear into constructive action.

Excess fear that doesn't result in corrective action, on the other hand, can only upset you and be harmful for your baby. The most effective way to cancel fearful thoughts is through *positive affirmations,* a form of positive thinking. Affirming positive thoughts creates bodily sensations of openness and expansiveness; that is, they relax your body. You can use these affirmations throughout the day to convert stressful, negative thoughts into positive actions. Affirmations actually transform your brain waves from alert, panicky delta waves into more relaxed alpha waves—which is why they are called *psychocatalyzers* in some yoga schools.

You can use several of the following affirmations throughout your pregnancy, labor, and childbirth. Sit or lie down on your back in a comfortable position, begin abdominal breathing, and, as you inhale, say the affirmation out loud.

**Pregnancy Affirmations**

*I am calm and relaxed.*

*The baby feels my calmness and shares it.*

*The baby and I are rested and ready for the work we will do.*

**Labor Affirmations**

*With each contraction, my cervix is dilating more and more, and the baby is descending.*

*The contractions of my uterus are massaging the baby, hugging it.*

*My belly feels as if it's suspended in warm water, floating lightly.*

*My breathing is slow and even.*

*My legs, hands, face, shoulders, stomach, and abdomen are relaxed. My belly and pelvis feel relaxed.*

*I am open, open, open.*

**Childbirth Affirmations**

*The baby is descending naturally. With each contraction, the baby descends a little more.*

*Soon my baby will be here.*

*The baby and I are doing beautifully.*

*My vagina stretches as the baby's head crowns, then emerges. I think of coolness, coolness.*

*Now the baby is here. My baby is beautiful.*

## Progressive Relaxation Exercises

Progressive relaxation is another effective method for inducing the relaxation response. Basically, it involves gently tensing (contracting) a muscle group—such as your back and neck muscles—for a few seconds, then relaxing them. You then repeat the technique for your neck, upper chest, arms, abdomen, hips, buttocks, thighs, knees, calves, and feet. A complete series of exercises produces a deep state of relaxation.

Follow these simple steps.

1.  Lie on your back and imagine your body sinking into the ground.

2.  Lift your left leg about a foot off the ground. Flex your foot and contract your leg muscles for five to ten seconds, then lower your leg to the floor and feel it relax.

3. Repeat the exercise for the right leg.

4. Tense your shoulders, then relax.

5. Tense your arms, then relax.

6. When you've completed two repetitions for the legs, shoulders, and arms, take a deep breath and slowly stand up and stretch. You should feel totally renewed.

## White-Light Visualization

Visualization is another excellent way of inducing the relaxation response and creating positive, pleasurable images about childbirth. Visualization, like receptive and guided imagery, takes advantage of the body's inability to distinguish between imagined (thought) events and actual events. The following visualization technique is taught in the Dick-Read pregnancy classes. It's designed for women in the advanced stages of pregnancy and labor, but it's useful throughout your entire pregnancy.

1. Sit or lie in a comfortable position with your eyes closed.

2. Breathe slowly and deeply. As you inhale, visualize your breath as a radiant white light filling your body.

3. As you exhale, imagine the light passing out of your body through the soles of your feet, carrying the tension away.

4. Repeat step 3 as many times as needed, directing the light to each part of your body.

5. Enjoy the feeling of complete relaxation for a few minutes.

6. Take one last deep breath, open your eyes, and stretch.

You can use this visualization as a mini-relaxer throughout the day. Whenever you feel tension, fatigue, or anxiety, try to stop what you're doing and imagine a white light filling your body. It's very important for you to be comfortable during your visualization. Experiment with variations in your breathing and find the visual image that helps you relax the most. You may also find that combining visualization with alternate-nostril breathing heightens your visualization.

## Receptive Imagery

Receptive imagery is a type of visualization that involves relaxing and letting any subconscious images you might have about being pregnant rise to the surface. Most pregnant women worry at some point during their pregnancy about their diet or if they're exercising enough. These anxieties are normal and can be helpful. They are best resolved, however, when you schedule fifteen minutes a day to meditate receptively on them, with the goal of taking practical steps at the end of your meditation to ensure you're doing everything possible to have a perfect birthing experience.

You can do this by combining your breathing exercises with a meditation in which you observe images and thoughts that just come to your mind. For example, you might meditate briefly on subjects such as nutrition, your exercise regimen, or preparations for the baby's arrival that you've been worrying about.

## Programmed Imagery

Choosing and holding specific images in your mind is called *programmed imagery*. You can use programmed imagery to enhance your relaxation during the last stages of labor. Programmed imagery is usually combined with affirmations. For example, the affirmation,

# Especially for Fathers

YOU MAY COME HOME FROM WORK THIS MONTH and find your partner meditating—and think she's joined an ashram! Don't panic: she's just doing one of the many relaxation exercises in this chapter. Why don't you join her? The exercises are really delightful and will further enhance the unity of your new family.

This trimester will be the most enjoyable for your partner. As her body adjusts to being pregnant, she'll feel better and her normal energy level will return. If you notice she's uncomfortable, take the initiative and suggest holistic ways to relieve her symptoms. If she's tired, try to take over more than your usual share of household chores, such as preparing meals or cleaning the house. One really helpful thing you can do is to make sure there are no dangerous toxins in the house, which are potentially dangerous for her or the baby. It's a big responsibility, and it will be a load off her shoulders.

"the muscles surrounding my uterus are relaxed," could be combined with deep breathing and a mental picture of your muscles relaxing. The affirmation image can physiologically relax the uterus and mentally alter your perception so that you feel less pain and work with your contractions.

Programmed imagery is very beneficial throughout your pregnancy and prior to labor. If you've had an upsetting day or your back aches, you'll find the following exercise very helpful in trying to relax, and in converting fearful thoughts into positive affirmations.

1.  Sit or lie down in a comfortable position and close your eyes.

2.  Breathe in and out deeply, allowing your abdomen to rise and fall.

3.  Imagine the relaxation in your whole body deepening by stages. You're now in a state in which your mind is clear and tranquil.

4.  Visualize yourself during childbirth. In the first visualization, imagine yourself having a relaxed, effortless, uncomplicated labor. In the second, visualize yourself being relaxed, focused, and joyful during the delivery of your baby.

## $\mathcal{H}$OLISTIC APPROACHES TO COMMON FOURTH-MONTH CONCERNS

Hemorrhoids, nasal congestion, and nosebleeds are common during the middle months of pregnancy and can be quite painful. Here are several holistic remedies designed to prevent or relieve them.

### Hemorrhoids

Fifty percent of all pregnant women develop *hemorrhoids,* which are varicose veins of the rectum. Pregnancy-induced constipation, lack of fiber and/or water in the diet, and insufficient exercise (especially Kegel exercises), are the most common causes of hemorrhoids. Sometimes rectal bleeding accompanies them. If your rectum starts to bleed, see your physician immediately. Hemorrhoids that appear as swellings and do not bleed may respond to the following holistic regimens.

### *Exercise*

Kegel exercises help prevent hemorrhoids (see Chapter 4). They strengthen the lower pelvic wall and rectum and increase blood flow and circulation so that blood doesn't pool in the rectal area.

*Homeopathy*  Homeopathic remedies, such as Silicea, Arsen alb., Lachesis, Acidum nit., *Calendula,* and hamamelis, have been used to treat hemorrhoids. Your caregiver or homeopath should recommend appropriate dosages.

*Hydrotherapy*  A warm bath at a temperature of 100°F is effective for hemorrhoids. Ice packs also reduce pain and swelling.

## Internal Hemorrhoids

Some women develop hemorrhoids higher up in the rectum. Like external hemorrhoids, they are painful and may or may not bleed. Normally, they are caused by constipation. They can be partially relieved by drinking lots of fluids, which keeps your stools soft. Unfortunately, there are no ointments that you can apply, because they are internal. They will heal eventually, especially if you use the nutritional remedies for rectal hemorrhoids. Sometimes they develop during the pushing in the second stage of labor.

## Vaginal Discharge

Slight spotting is common in early pregnancy and may occur when your period would normally be due, after making love, or as a result of a vaginal infection. You may also notice a slight increase in monthly white discharges. This occurs in most pregnant women, because glands in the walls of the vagina secrete more mucus. This extra discharge is unlikely to affect your baby. You should bring persistent leakage to your caregiver's attention, however, because it may be a sign of a deficiency in B vitamins, in which case your caregiver may recommend supplements.

Dark or bright red blood should be brought to your caregiver's attention immediately. Sometimes the bleeding will stop after bed rest with no harm to the fetus, and your pregnancy can continue. Ask your caregiver what measures to take to strengthen your ability to sustain your pregnancy.

*Douching*  Gentle douching with water, vinegar and water, or a water-soluble lubricant such as K-Y jelly (provided it doesn't cause any irritation) will help reduce heavier secretions. Different caregivers have different rules about douching. Some recommend that you not douche at all because it often removes helpful bacterial in the vagina. The best advice is to douche only when it is strongly recommended by your caregiver to treat a persistent problem, such as a heavy vaginal discharge. Be sure to use only disposable douches and low water pressure.

Remember, your husband or partner must also maintain strict hygiene, as most vaginal infections that arise during pregnancy are caused by bacteria transmitted by the partner's fingers, penis, or mouth.

*Homeopathy*

Natrum Phosphoricum 6X tissue salts, taken three times daily for a week, are given to help stabilize any acid/alkaline imbalance and decrease vaginal secretions. This remedy should be prescribed by a homeopath and approved by your caregiver.

*Nutrition and Supplements*

Excessive vaginal secretions can also be caused by a poor diet, particularly by the overconsumption of refined sugar-rich foods. To reverse the symptoms, follow the dietary guidelines for relieving cramping (see Chapter 5). Increase your intake of green leafy vegetables (except cabbage and Brussels sprouts, if they give you gas) and fish. Alcohol, tobacco, coffee, tea, chocolate, and other caffeine-containing foods and beverages should also be restricted. Another way to balance alkaline and acid levels is to drink one teaspoon of apple cider vinegar in eight ounces of water several times daily. This helps balance acid/alkaline levels in stomach and vaginal secretions.

# Nasal Congestion

Nasal congestion, usually accompanied by an occasional nosebleed, is a common complaint during pregnancy, probably because the high levels of estrogen and progesterone circulating in the blood increase blood flow to the mucous membranes of the nose, causing them to soften and swell—just as the cervix does in preparation for childbirth. Congestion and bleeding are more common during the winter, when heating systems force hot, dry air into the house, drying delicate nasal passages. It's best not to use any medications or nasal sprays, unless they are prescribed by your caregiver. A humidifier helps overcome nasal dryness, and lubricating each nostril with a dab of petroleum jelly will relieve some of the symptoms.

*Acupuncture*

Acupuncture effectively relieves nasal congestion by stimulating detoxification of the body, which allows its resistance to histamines (the cause of congestion) to improve. Once this happens, nasal congestion is usually alleviated within minutes, and the relief usually lasts for several weeks.

*Acupressure*

You can also use self-acupressure to relieve minor nasal congestion that's not caused by allergies. Place your thumbs on the outer portion of your upper chest and press on the muscles that run horizontally below your collarbone. You should feel a sensitive spot (or knot) on your chest muscles. Under that knot is *LU1,* an important acupressure point for relieving breathing difficulties. Let your head hang forward toward your chest and relax your neck as you maintain firm pressure on those muscles with your thumbs. Continue to hold these points while you breathe deeply for two minutes.

*Aromatherapy*

To relieve nasal congestion during an asthma-like attack, inhale an infusion made of bergamot, camphor, eucalyptus, lavender, hyssop, or marjoram. Frankincense has also been used to relieve congestion and help relax pregnant women. Inhaling an infusion of vapor rub is also helpful.

*Ayurvedic Medicine*

Drink a tea made from a half teaspoon of licorice and ginger dissolved in a cup of water. (Women with high blood pressure should avoid consuming licorice or teas made with licorice because of its hypertensive effect.) To further relieve congestion and coughing, try a quarter cup of onion juice with a teaspoon of honey and an eighth teaspoon of black pepper. For sneezing, try ashwagandha, shatavari, gotu kola, and triphala.

*Botanical Medicines*

Taking anise oil (the active ingredients of thyme) mixed with honey before each meal will help your body break up and eliminate lung secretions. Comfrey, fennel seed, fenugreek, licorice root, rose hips, and rosemary have similar beneficial effects.

*Hydrotherapy*

Hot and cold packs placed on the chest and abdomen may relieve some forms of nasal congestion. Sine-wave electrical pads can also be used to stimulate the nervous system to clear the nasal passage. Wet hot compresses (be sure to wring them out) of folded flannel cloth applied across the forehead and sinus may also help ease symptoms.

*Nutrition and Supplements*

The best diet to alleviate nasal congestion is a very light one emphasizing fruits and vegetable broths. Avoid concentrated sugars, because they slow down immune function and encourage bacterial activity. Also, avoid foods to which you've developed allergies or sensitivities. Be sure to fully digest all your food during meals. Stress control is also crucial.

Vitamin and mineral supplements can also relieve nasal congestion. Ask your caregiver about your need for vitamin A or beta carotene, vitamin B$_5$, vitamin C, vitamin E, zinc, selenium, N-acetyl cysteine (an amino acid), or essential fatty acids (in the form of evening primrose oil, black currant oil, or flaxseed oil).

## Nosebleeds

Occasional nosebleeds are not dangerous. They are usually caused simply by blowing your nose too hard or fingernail scratches. Recurring nose bleeds, however, may be a result of high blood pressure (hypertension), so be sure to consult your caregiver about them.

Taking the RDA for vitamin K can help prevent nosebleeds. The fastest way to relieve a minor nosebleed is to squeeze the contents of vitamin E and vitamin A capsules into the lining of your nose. You may also use zinc oxide, petroleum jelly, aloe vera gel, comfrey, or calendula ointment, then place small pieces of gauze inside. Midwives caution against using baby oils, and recommend instead using an all-natural oil, such as primrose oil. Some women will find that they can stop nosebleeds by applying ice packs to the nose.

### Aromatherapy

Inhaling lemon, lavender, cypress, or frankincense infusions may help stop periodic nosebleeds.

### Nutrition and Supplements

Sometimes the natural flora of pregnant women does not make enough vitamin K, which is essential for blood clotting and helps prevent nosebleeds. Midwives have found that eating foods rich in vitamin K—such as watercress, dark green leafy vegetables, kale, and alfalfa—helps prevent nosebleeds.

Taking 3 grams of vitamin C at the start of a nosebleed may eliminate nosebleeds in some women. Most nosebleeds will stop after a short period of time. But if they don't, be sure to call your caregiver. Rutin and other bioflavonoids are also helpful. Ask your holistic caregiver to prescribe appropriate dosages.

Twelve breathing exercises, three visualizations, laughter, meditation—you might think you're in an advanced yoga class—but these are all simple, enjoyable, and essential components of the Holistic Pregnancy Program to keep you relaxed and confident. You'll find yourself going through the day with a sparkling grin on your face. Happiness is contagious. So, to infect yourself with good vibes, put yourself in its way!

## Chapter 6

# The Fifth Month

*T*HIS MONTH IS GOING TO BE REALLY THRILLING FOR YOU! During this month's checkup, you will probably be able to hear your baby's heartbeat for the first time. After hearing those precious little thumps, you're likely to look forward to your baby's birth with renewed excitement and energy.

Your baby is now about ten inches long and growing by leaps and bounds, using the hands to grip and the eyelids starting to blink. The bones inside the ears (the *auditory ossicles*) have hardened, so now your baby can hear! You might even notice that your baby seems to move when you play loud music (not a good idea). Your child is really beginning to take on an identity.

In this chapter, we'll concentrate on ways to keep feeling and looking good.

## *T*HE FIFTH-MONTH CHECKUP

One of the joys of this month's checkup will be counting your baby's heartbeats with an ordinary stethoscope or fetoscope. Make a special effort to take your partner with you to this appointment—this is a moment that is not to be missed.

During this visit, your caregiver will also monitor your weight and blood pressure, take a urine sample, evaluate the size and position of your uterus and the height of your fundus, look for signs of edema and varicose veins, and evaluate any unusual symptoms you're experiencing.

You may find that your baby's growth and movements inside your womb cause insomnia, swelling (edema) of your feet and ankles, or varicose veins. This chapter discusses several holistic remedies for these discomforts. You may want to discuss them with your caregiver during this month's checkup. This is also a good time to discuss immunizations for yourself and your baby, if you haven't already done so.

## COMMON FIFTH-MONTH CONCERNS

### Immunizations

Sometimes vaccination dilemmas arise during pregnancy, and you need to know how to deal with them. Four common types of immunizing agents are used in the United States and Canada: live virus vaccines, inactive bacterial vaccines, viral vaccines, and immunoglobulin preparations.

You should only have vaccinations that your caregiver recommends to protect you and your baby. As a precaution, avoid traveling to areas where certain infectious disorders, such as plague or yellow fever, are common. If you're a teacher and you're not already immune, stay home if epidemics of rubella, influenza, or chickenpox break out in your school.

### Making Love

Sex during pregnancy can be wonderful. There's nothing like the warmth of physical and emotional intimacy to help you feel relaxed and healthy.

Many women find pregnancy a sexually erotic time, but worry that lovemaking may injure their baby. You need not be concerned— orgasm is both safe and beneficial, because it stimulates your uterus and prepares your body for birth. Your growing baby is well protected by the amniotic membranes and fluids, and deep penetration will not harm it since your uterus is located well above the vagina.

In most cases, vaginal penetration is perfectly safe as long as you're not experiencing vaginal bleeding or a vaginal infection. Your caregiver may advise against sexual intercourse if you have a history of incompetent cervical closure or premature rupturing of membranes (PROM). You may also be advised to avoid vaginal penetration for the first four or five months, until your pregnancy is well established, if you have a tendency to miscarry. Vaginal penetration may be difficult late in pregnancy if the baby's head is deep in your pelvis. At that time, you and your partner should explore other forms of sexual gratification—for example, taking herbal baths together, then giving each other an erotic massage. Nipple massage is an excellent way to prepare your breasts for breastfeeding. It's also normal to masturbate.

Occasionally lovemaking is followed by slightly pink spotting, because the blood vessels around the cervix are more plentiful during pregnancy and some may rupture. This is usually not a cause for concern, although it's a good idea to inform your caregiver, who may recommend that you avoid deep penetration for awhile.

Some women find that their uterus remains hard for several minutes after orgasm or contracts in short spasms. These contractions are normal. They are called Braxton-Hicks contractions, and they occur more frequently toward the end of pregnancy as the uterus prepares for birth. Most Braxton-Hicks contractions, however, occur spontaneously, and only in rare cases after intercourse. If you find that intercourse stimulates consistent contractions, report this to your caregiver.

From mid-pregnancy on, it's a good idea not to lie on your stomach with your weight on the baby. Lying on your side during sex, with your partner behind you, may be more comfortable and allows you to control the depth of penetration. You can also kneel with your stomach supported by a pile of cushions, while your partner enters from behind.

Keep in mind that you're at slightly greater risk of contracting a variety of infectious diseases, such as herpes (see below), while you're pregnant. It's extremely important that you and your partner be tested to make sure you're not infected with any viruses, which—along with liver infections (avoid eating undercooked meat), kidney damage, and malnutrition—put your baby at risk and can cause premature labor and stillbirth. Your caregiver should monitor you carefully for these complications throughout your pregnancy.

# ESPECIALLY for FATHERS

AS YOUR PARTNER'S ABDOMEN GROWS, her pregnancy will become more obvious to you and to others. She may actually be able to feel the fetus move and soon you will, too, with your hand on her abdomen. Both of you should be able to hear your child's heartbeat during this month's checkup.

One really helpful thing you can do this month is to understand the physical changes your partner is going through. She may feel uncomfortable because of her weight gain and the change in her body shape. It's your job to take over more of the household duties to give her a chance to get accustomed to these changes and appreciate them.

You can also show her how much you appreciate her with a small, meaningful gift or by surprising her with one of the massages we recommend. You should also encourage her to pamper herself. An evening "off" with friends or time alone to curl up with a good book, to "surf the net" without interruption, or to explore the town, or go for a walk will help her appreciate her pregnancy (and you!)—and relax.

# HOLISTIC BEAUTY PROGRAM

Pregnancy is a time to take special care of yourself—to make sure you get enough sleep and exercise, eat properly, and pamper yourself. You may have noticed that even if you haven't gained a significant amount of weight, you can't button your skirts and your blouses and bras are uncomfortable. Your muscles have started to stretch in preparation for changes that will occur later. At times, you may feel overweight and uncomfortable.

You need to remind yourself that while you're gaining weight, you're storing protection for your baby. Purchase clothes you like that fit properly or borrow items from friends, relatives, and even your partner's closet. Consider enrolling in a prenatal exercise class. Feeling good about your appearance may help you feel more confident.

## Skin Care

Some women find that pregnancy enhances their skin tone, while others find that they will need to constantly massage their skin to help bring more oils to the surface. Natural body oils help maintain the natural suppleness of the skin. If you had healthy, vibrant skin before your pregnancy, chances are you will continue to have it throughout your pregnancy.

### *Facial Care*

You can keep your skin naturally healthy by using herbal scrubs, masks, lotions, and moisturizers. For your face, try gentle, non-abrasive scrubs, lotions, and moisturizers—oatmeal scrubs, for example, are very gentle for most skin textures. Use your fingertips, not a washcloth, to gently apply the scrub for fifteen to thirty seconds.

If you have dry, sensitive skin, apply facial scrubs very lightly, and stop when your skin becomes slightly flushed. Then rinse with water, dry the skin, and apply a natural moisturizer. Clay-based facial masks are excellent for removing dead cells and excess surface oil. Bentonite clay masks may help eliminate acne. Once you remove the mask, rub vitamin E oil on your skin. Some women let the oil remain on their skin for thirty minutes, then apply a coating of whisked egg whites (which contain protein) over the vitamin E oil. Rinse the coating off with filtered water.

If clay dries your skin too much, try a natural clay mask made with fruit enzymes, such as papain (from papaya) or bromelain (from pineapple) which are now available in health food stores. You can also make your own moisturizer by combining one tablespoon of almond oil with three tablespoons of avocado oil and one teaspoon of beeswax. Stir until creamy, let cool, and apply with your fingers.

If you like, you can also make your own skin toner by boiling a cup of lilac leaves in two cups of water, simmering it for ten minutes, and letting it cool for several hours. Then strain the mixture and apply several drops to your face and neck with a sterile pad.

You can make your own hand cream by adding equal amounts of rose water and milk to cooked, peeled potatoes in a bowl, then adding two drops of glycerine and mixing into a paste.

For flaky lips, try one of the new herbal lip masks, moisturizers, or emollients. They can be used before applying your lipstick.

Avoid spending too much time in the sun; if you must, be sure to use a natural sun block. If you get sunburned, immediately apply aloe vera gel directly to your skin.

## Hair Care

During pregnancy, your hair is likely to feel fuller and healthier than before. You can continue your usual hair-care routine, but don't use any dyes or chemicals. Avoid perms; use rollers, pin curls, teasing, or nonchemical straighteners instead. Also, avoid metal-based hair dyes; use natural dyes, such as henna, instead. It's best to use natural-bristle hairbrushes and keep vigorous brushing to a minimum. Natural brushes help distribute the oils in your hair better and don't stress the follicles as much.

Pregnancy sometimes straightens curls, and your hair may become drier. Try an all-herbal shampoo and conditioner to keep your hair looking healthy. A quick head and neck massage is a great way to loosen scalp flakes and stimulate circulation, which is important for healthy hair growth. In the shower, with shampoo in your hair, move the balls of your fingers in little circles over the entire scalp. Start at the front, just below the hairline, and move backwards, using both hands, with fingers spread apart. Lift your fingers (don't drag them) each time you move to another spot. Don't forget the base of your skull and the back of your neck.

After rinsing out the shampoo, apply a natural hair conditioner, if you like. You can make your own conditioner by mixing a half cup of rosemary oil with one and a half ounces of sweet almond oil and ten drops of orange oil extract.

### Body Hair

During pregnancy, hormonal changes sometimes cause body hair to grow faster than normal. If you're lucky, you'll end up with thicker and more lustrous hair on your head. The downside, however, is that pregnancy can also stimulate hair growth in places where you wish it didn't—especially your lips, chin, cheeks, arms, legs, back, and belly. Most of this excess hair will disappear within six months postpartum. The least stressful way to handle this situation is to ignore it. If you can't, then try plucking, shaving, or using a natural depilatory or cream recommended by your caregiver.

## Breast Care

In addition to swelling, you may find that your breasts develop dark patches and bumps. The dark pigmented area around your nipples—

called the *areolae*—may become even darker, but usually lightens after birth. The little bumps you may notice on the areolae are *sebaceous glands;* that is, they secrete an oily lubricating liquid. These glands become more prominent during pregnancy but usually will return to their normal size once your baby is born.

By the fifth month, your breasts may also begin secreting a thick, yellowish liquid called *colostrum,* an antibody-rich fluid that will nourish your baby until your milk comes in, when your baby is born. If it cakes on your breasts, you can soften and remove the colostrum with warm water. If it gets too thick, very gentle pressure with the thumb and forefinger at the base of the nipple will clear the little openings into the breast.

It's a good idea to massage your nipples daily with natural safflower and almond oil creams, especially if you plan to breastfeed. The massage helps stimulate milk production. After bathing, rub each nipple gently with a soft terry cloth towel, then place a thumb and forefinger near the base of the nipple and press gently together. Draw the nipple outward, and turn it up and down. Do this several times with each nipple. If the nipple is slightly retracted and doesn't stand erect, consult your caregiver. In addition to nipple pulling, you may be advised to wear a breast shield to help your nipples protrude. The nipples need to protrude for your baby to breastfeed.

## Clothes

There's never been a more fashionable time to be pregnant. Many department stores now offer maternity clothes in attractive styles which are very comfortable and practical and can be worn in even the most corporate of offices. Ask a lingerie salesperson to help you choose a bra and other maternity underwear that fit well and are comfortable.

Remember that your body temperature will increase during pregnancy, so you may feel more comfortable in fabrics that breathe, like cotton. Light colors, mesh weaves, and loose garments will also help keep you cool. You'll probably find knee-highs more comfortable than panty hose, but avoid those that have narrow, constrictive bands at the top, as they can increase your risk for varicose veins and irritate your skin. When the weather turns cold, dress in layers to draw sweat away from the body and so that you can selectively peel them off as you heat up or go indoors.

# Holistic Approaches to Common Fifth-Month Concerns

Acne

Acne blemishes are usually due to hormonal changes and usually clear up by the last trimester. You don't have to wait until then, however. You might be able to speed up Mother Nature with the holistic remedies described below.

*Botanical Medicines*

Steaming your face with botanical infusions of bergamot, lavender, rosemary, or rosewood may help clear up acne. A facial-scrub massage with bergamot, camphor, geranium, juniper, or lavender will clean facial pores and eliminate acne debris. Ayurvedic herbs—such as neroli, tumeric, or sandalwood—are also helpful in cleaning pores.

Chamomile preparations are widely used in Europe to treat acne and other skin problems. Tea tree oil is as effective as benzyl peroxide in reversing acne and has no side effects. Aloe vera gel may also relieve acne.

*Homeopathy*

According to Dana Ullmans' *Discovering Homeopathy: Medicine for the 21st Century,* homeopathic remedies—including pulsatilla, silicea, *Berberis,* Ledum, sulfur, Arsen alb., and belladonna—have proven effective in clinical trials in reversing common acne.

*Hydrotherapy*

Some women find that applying lukewarm or cold water to their face throughout the day clears up acne. Midwives also recommend taking hot Epsom salts baths two to three times a week. This safely relieves acne on the face and other skin irritations around the breasts or on the legs.

*Nutrition and Supplements*

Some women find that their acne improves if they stop eating certain foods, such as chocolate, fruit juices, carbonated beverages, caffeinated beverages, or milk and milk products. Excessive long-term consumption of seafood or other foods rich in iodine may also cause acne outbreaks in some women. A good anti-acne food plan includes four to five servings of raw vegetables. Some holistic caregivers believe that excessive consumption of animal fats causes acne, and that switching to a vegetable-rich diet reduces outbreaks.

Make sure that you consume the RDAs for zinc, selenium, and vitamin E, because these nutrients may help prevent acne. Vitamin $B_6$ also prevents acne, although supplementation may be necessary.

If you also have gum problems, ask your caregiver if you would benefit from taking folic acid supplements.

## Rash

Some mothers-to-be also develop pinpoint rashes on their chest, abdomen, and back. These are sometimes caused by additives in iron supplements, so be sure to take only natural iron supplements.

*Ayurvedic Medicine*

Several Ayurvedic formulas relieve skin rashes effectively. Try applying the pulp of the cilantro leaf to the rash or drinking two tablespoons of fresh cilantro tea three times daily. Tea made with one cup water, one teaspoon coriander seeds, a pinch of black pepper, and a half teaspoon of ghee (clarified butter) is also helpful. Also, neem oil can be applied topically.

*Botanical Medicine*

Burdock root or gentian root supplements have been used to eliminate skin rashes. Fresh coriander or flavored aloe vera juice may also be beneficial.

*Homeopathy*

Ask your homeopath about taking belladonna, sulfur, or graphites to reverse skin rashes.

*Hydrotherapy*

A warm bath containing one tablespoon of baking soda is useful for relieving the itch caused by most skin rashes. You can also try soaking in a lukewarm bath to which a cup of oatmeal has been added.

*Nutrition and Supplements*

Food allergies or sensitivities can cause a skin rash. Try eating more fresh green leafy vegetables and restricting your intake of citrus fruits, berries, peanuts, shellfish, and milk and milk products. Taking a half teaspoon of baking soda in water every few hours may eliminate some rashes.

You may find that flaxseed oil, eicosapentanoic acid (EPA), or gamma linolenic acid (GLA) supplements prevent skin rashes. Ask your caregiver if you would benefit from taking vitamin A, C, or E supplements or using skin lotions that contain these vitamins.

## Stretch Marks

Sometimes women develop stretch marks (*striae*), which are pigmented, itchy lines that develop on your breasts and abdomen. Many women appear to be genetically predisposed to developing striae.

While some women can gain sixty pounds without developing any marks, for others, a weight gain of ten pounds in two months will result in very deeply pigmented marks. Contrary to popular myths, stretch marks are not caused by losing weight. In fact, the opposite is true. They appear because the top layer of skin cannot grow quickly enough to encompass the added body mass, and stretch marks appear on the underlying skin level.

Stretch marks usually become much lighter and much less noticeable after childbirth. However, they may not disappear completely. You can minimize them with a holistic program that emphasizes (1) gaining a moderate amount of weight gradually and (2) massaging your breasts and abdomen daily with aloe vera and lanolin or almond oil.

You should start your stretch marks prevention routine before your skin begins to stretch. It's usually most convenient to massage in the morning when you wake up and just before bed at night. Try aloe vera, lanolin or almond oil, cocoa butter, or vitamin E lotions or gels. These are available at health food stores.

## Dry, Itchy Skin

You may develop dry skin, especially on the hands, knees, and feet during your pregnancy. This is due to genetics or exposure to forced hot air, too much sun, or irritating soap products that take too much oil out of your skin. The best way to remoisturize dry skin is to bathe in lukewarm water and use natural, unscented soaps. Always dry yourself gently after a bath, patting your skin to avoid chapping, and apply a natural moisturizing cream while your skin is still moist. Drinking lots of water and using humidifiers also helps.

### *Botanical Medicine*

Herbal moisturizing creams and facial masks that contain lavender, evening primrose, wheat germ, or chamomile may also help repair dry skin. Don't use lanolin lotions (which are made from sheep) if you're allergic to wool, because they can cause contact dermatitis.

## Oily Skin

Try using masks made of clay such as kaolin or Fuller's earth (available in most pharmacies or health food stores) to control the oil content on your face. You can make your own mask by combining a teaspoon of clay with enough water to make a paste. Allow the mask to dry on your face for ten minutes before rinsing it off with filtered water, witch hazel, diluted lemon juice, or a solution made of one part rubbing alcohol and ten parts water. Soaps containing *Calendula* may also help clean the pores without irritating the skin.

You might also try massaging your face in the morning and evening with a mixture of vitamin A emulsion, chlorophyll, aloe vera gel, or cider vinegar mixed with a dash of cayenne pepper. Some women massage their skin with an herbal tea consisting of a teaspoon of alfalfa, burdock root, echinacea, apple cider vinegar, and a dash of cayenne pepper.

## Chloasma

Some women develop *chloasma* (mask of pregnancy), a mottled darkening of the skin that usually is most obvious on the forehead, nose, and cheeks below the eyes. You may also notice some darkened tissue spreading from your pubic area upwards over your stomach. Aloe vera gel may help lighten these areas during pregnancy. Some women find that rubbing a piece of sliced red onion over the affected areas has the same effect. Darkened skin usually returns to its normal color after childbirth.

Some dark spots are caused by rubbing and irritation, usually on the arms or lower back of the neck. The best way to prevent these is to use a botanical cream that nourishes the skin so you won't have to scratch and subsequently reinjure it.

If you're a sun worshipper, you can prevent dark spots by using natural sunscreens. Better yet, limit the sunbathing. It's also important to refrain from smoking, which contributes to the breakdown of the skin's elasticity. Some medications also make the skin more fragile. You are more likely to develop darks spots, for example, if you use aspirin regularly, take oral prednisone, or use strong topical steroid creams.

## Herpes

You should find out, as early in pregnancy as possible, whether you have herpes. Two types of herpes simplex virus (HSV) are common: HSV-I (oral herpes) and HSV-II (genital herpes). *Oral herpes* is an infectious cold sore which usually appears on the lips or nostrils, although it can be spread to the genitals by oral sex. It usually dries up, if left alone, in five to ten days.

## OTHER SKIN PROBLEMS

Red dots. Sometimes little red dots appear on the neck and arms early in pregnancy and seem to gradually increase in size. They are not very noticeable and usually disappear after the baby is born.

Scars. You may find that you scar more easily when you're pregnant. This is usually due to a nutritional deficiency. You should mention it to your holistic caregiver if the scars don't disappear.

Psoriasis. Red, scaly skin on the elbows or knees may indicate psoriasis. Don't scratch the scales, as this can irritate the skin. Instead, ask your caregiver or dermatologist to identify the causes and prescribe remedies to relieve them.

Dermatitis. Scaly red patches may grow on your eyebrows and the sides of your nose. These may be caused by reactions to fabric softeners and detergents, dog or cat fur, or deodorizers. To prevent dermatitis, use natural unscented detergents, avoid petting animals, and wear garments with long sleeves when working outdoors. Once the irritant is removed, use a botanical cream lotion. Try to wash the area with a mild, soap-free cleanser, and use a natural moisturizer containing licorice, which is a safer and more effective option than cortisone cream lotions. If the flakes don't disappear after two weeks, see a dermatologist.

*Genital herpes* is transmitted through sexual contact. It usually breaks out on the genitals, although transmission can occur on any body surface that makes contact with an active herpes sore, in the mouth through oral-genital sexual contact or anywhere the infected person auto-inoculates herself (for example, by touching an active sore on the mouth and later touching the genitals). There is no cure for HSV-II; once you get it, you'll have it forever.

You can, by the way, have both types of herpes at the same time. The danger of both types is the same: they attack and weaken your immune system. The symptoms include fever and excruciating pain in the joints; the sores are actually secondary symptoms. You can get either type of herpes from your partner. In males, the sores usually appear as tiny, pinpoint blisters on the penis or foreskin. Ask your caregiver for medication if you notice that your partner has these sores.

Some people are asymptomatic—that is, they do not develop lesions, but they have the virus, anyway. One symptom is a tingling, burning sensation around a cold sore, either on the genital area or on the mouth. Remember, oral herpes sores can break out on the genitals, and genital herpes sores can appear as cold sores on the face. By the time the tingling starts, the virus is already active. Even if you have it on your buttocks, it can still infect your cervix.

Herpes tests (called cultures) take four to five days to come back from the laboratory, by which time your symptoms may have disappeared—that is, you may not have obvious sores. You may still have active herpes, however. You need to be examined externally for lesions and internally for infected genitalia. If, during labor, your caregiver determines that your membranes are intact, you may be able to have a vaginal delivery. If you have active herpes, however, your caregiver will probably recommend a cesarean delivery because of the risk of death and blindness for babies delivered vaginally to herpes-infected mothers.

**Botanical Medicine**

Depending on the type of sores you have, there are several botanical supplements you can take. Lemon, geranium, eucalyptus, and bergamot oils are antiseptics that are applied to the skin at the first sign of an outbreak to relieve HSV-1 flare-ups. Rose, melissa, lavender, and tea tree oils are also effective. Ask your caregiver which of these is best to relieve your symptoms.

Echinacea, licorice, pokeweed, lentinus edodes (a mushroom extract), and Cat's Claw (a woody vine that grows in Peru) have been used to relieve the pain of herpes genitalis. These can be taken as capsules or made into teas. Some symptoms can also be relieved with wild oat, boxweed, burdock, and garlic supplements. You can also try applying a lotion of dwarf nettle and *Calendula* to the sores. Inserting a small muslin bag filled with finely crushed garlic into the vagina shortens some herpes infection cycles. This is safe and effective, and should not be painful. If you find it uncomfortable, try a smaller bag. The bag should be left in place for four to six hours, and should be removed if it causes burning. Garlic is an antiseptic and poses no risk to the fetus.

Apply herbal compresses of aloe, goldenseal, and lavender directly to lesions to relieve itching. Topical ointments containing licorice root, lithium succinate, and zinc have also been used to relieve herpes.

Cuban physicians have treated herpes effectively with ozone water mixed with sunflower oil and applied externally. Ozone-enriched water is now available in some health food stores.

**Homeopathy**

Natrum muriaticum or *Rhus* toxicodendron taken three times daily for three days has also helped some women reverse the symptoms of oral herpes infections.

**Baths**

Ask your caregiver about the advisability of taking an herbal bath to relieve symptoms of herpes. Sitting in mildly hot (98°F) bath water containing one cup of chamomile tea and ten drops of *Calendula* tincture can reduce symptoms. You can also try bathing in bath water containing a cup of Epsom salts. As noted, bathing in Epsom salts is safe and effectively relieves vaginal irritations, including herpes. Discontinue bathing if you notice any bleeding or vaginal irritations, and report them to your caregiver.

**Nutrition and Supplements**

Some herpes infections result from dietary imbalances or food allergies. A simple rotation elimination diet may help you identify foods that cause the outbreaks. Try replacing all simple sugars and refined foods with organic fruits, garlic, and onions, which may inhibit herpes flare-ups.

In addition, drink eight 8-ounce glasses of water every day. This will make your urine less acidic and ease the pain of urinating.

---

## PREVENTING HERPES INFECTIONS

You can prevent herpes infections by taking the following precautions:

▷ Avoid sexual contact altogether when lesions are active. Condoms do not guarantee safety.

▷ Avoid kissing your partner when blisters appear on either your lips or mouth.

▷ Don't share clothing, utensils, or other objects with an infected person.

▷ Always wash your hands before and after touching any part of your body or your partner's body.

Ask your caregiver to recommend appropriate doses of the beta carotene, vitamin C, pantothenic acid, and zinc supplements to relieve herpes. Lysine (an amino acid) supplements have also been used to prevent herpes outbreaks.

## Cramps

Some women experience menstrual-like cramps during pregnancy, especially after making love. These are usually triggered by a hormone *(oxytocin)* that makes the uterus contract. Occasional cramping of this type is usually not dangerous. If cramping continues for more than a week, however, discuss it with your caregiver.

You may also experience muscle cramps over the pubic bone when you cough or sneeze. These are not uterine cramps. There are two possible causes: (1) stretching of the *round ligaments,* which anchor your uterus within the pelvic cavity; and (2) softening of the pubic bone, which is a natural occurrence during pregnancy and which is more noticeable at five months or later, when the baby's hard head is pressing against the pubic bone. Try bending over before you cough or sneeze—this will move the baby upwards and reduce the pressure against your pubic bone. Acupuncture may also reduce cramping, especially if it is accompanied by chronic back pain and migraine headaches.

### Botanical Therapies

Ginger, white willow bark, red raspberry leaf, chamomile, hops, ginkgo biloba, and chaste tree berry supplements may help relieve cramps. Bromelain extract from pineapples has also been used to ease cramping. An herbalist will recommend the botanical medicine most appropriate for your symptoms.

### Nutrition and Supplements

In some cases, cramping is caused by diets that are high in fat and simple carbohydrates. Try eliminating simple carbohydrates (such as sugar, honey, white flour, maple syrup, dried fruit, and fruit juices) first. Cut down on saturated fats, too, replacing them with vegetable oils, which are rich in linoleic and linolenic acids. Replace red meat in your diet with other protein sources, such as fish or legumes, combined with whole grains (for example, beans and rice). Also, increase your intake of green leafy vegetables and restrict your intake of alcohol and tobacco, as well as coffee, tea, chocolate, and other foods and beverages with caffeine.

| | |
|---|---|
| ***Traditional Chinese Medicine (TCM)*** | According to TCM practitioners, cramps can also be caused by chi stagnation in the lower abdomen. Acupuncture and Chinese herbs administered by a licensed TCM practitioner may relieve symptoms by restoring a normal chi flow to your lower abdomen. |

## Moderately High Blood Pressure

Most women find that their blood pressure levels increase during pregnancy. Mild increases are considered normal. Your blood pressure will be measured during your monthly visits with your caregiver. The average blood pressure for healthy adults is 120/80. For women in their childbearing years, the average is often lower—between 100/60 and 110/70. These numbers represent the pressure created by the flow of blood through your veins under two circumstances. The first number is the *systolic blood pressure*—the pressure created when your heart is fully contracted. The second number is the *diastolic blood pressure,* and represents the pressure when your heart is at rest. Blood pressure may vary during pregnancy. Your caregiver will establish a baseline reading early in your pregnancy and to monitor your blood pressure each month. By having your pressure monitored regularly, you can catch any signs of pregnancy-induced hypertension (PIH) early, before it progresses to a more dangerous condition. Most women experience a decrease in blood pressure in their fifth or sixth month of pregnancy.

| | |
|---|---|
| ***Acupuncture*** | Some women develop moderately high blood pressure because of stress and difficulty sleeping. Acupuncture can reduce stress and relieve insomnia and, thus, lower blood pressure indirectly. Be sure to see an acupuncturist who specializes in treating pregnant women. |
| ***Biofeedback*** | A simple biofeedback exercise, in which you mentally focus on increasing the temperature of your fingers and hands, can lower your blood pressure. This exercise doesn't work for everyone, however. It has not been proven beneficial for women with extremely high blood pressure. |
| ***Botanical Medicines*** | Pacific oyster supplements (ask your caregiver about optimum dosages) are effective in reducing mildly elevated blood pressure in some women. Don't use them if you're allergic to shellfish, however. |

Passion flower and *Chlorella* (a genus of green algae that are high in beta carotene, iron, zinc, and vitamin B$_{12}$) also lower blood pressure and cholesterol levels. Maitake and reishi mushrooms and garlic supplements may also help.

***Physical Activity***

It might seem odd to lift five-pound weights three times a week to lower your blood pressure, but a Johns Hopkins study, cited in the May 1990 issue of the *Mayo Clinic Nutrition Letter,* found that weight lifting, walking, or jogging three times a week for twenty minutes each time reduced blood pressure by approximately six points.

***Mineral Salt Substitutes***

Another way of lowering moderately elevated blood pressure is by using mineral salt substitutes. In one study, Dutch physicians lowered the blood pressure in a group of 100 men and women with moderate hypertension by replacing table salt in their diets with low-sodium, high-potassium, high-magnesium mineral salts.

***Nutrition and Supplements***

A low-sodium diet may effectively lower your blood pressure. Normally, this means restricting your use of table salt, foods that contain large amounts of sodium, and laxatives and medicines (your caregiver can also advise you of the sodium content of prescription and over-the-counter medications). You should continue to eat lots of vegetables, whole grains, and fruits, and moderate amounts of milk and milk products and lean protein-rich foods every day. If you miss the taste of salt, try sprinkling lemon juice or vinegar on your foods.

If you decide to reduce your salt intake, try reducing your intake of canned, salted, or smoked meats, such as bacon, cold cuts, chipped or corned beef, frankfurters, ham, kosher meats, salt pork, or sausage. Also avoid salted nuts or nut butters and meat extracts, bouillon, and prepared soups.

Adding fiber to your daily diet can also help you keep your blood pressure under control.

***Tai Chi***

Tai chi, or moving meditation, can also help restore normal blood pressure levels. In a study reported in the May 1992 issue of the *Journal of Psychosomatic Research,* forty-eight women who practiced tai chi, brisk walking, and meditation lowered both their blood pressure and heart rate levels by 20 percent.

*Visualization*

Try meditation, relaxation, and visualization exercises to reduce your blood pressure. Sit calmly in a meditative pose, breathe deeply, and tell your heart to beat slower. This may lower your diastolic blood pressure. It usually takes ten to fifteen minutes for your blood pressure to drop.

*Nutrition and Supplements*

Dr. Dean Ornish's *Program for Reversing Heart Disease* suggests that taking magnesium supplements also reduces blood pressure. Low magnesium levels are often found in pregnant women with elevated blood pressure levels. Ask your caregiver to prescribe an appropriate dose.

# Pregnancy-Induced Hypertension (PIH)

If you have high blood pressure (140/90 or higher) accompanied by a reading of +1 on a urine dipstick and/or pitting edema (swollen tissue in which moderate finger pressure leaves an impression), blurred vision, or epigastric (near the stomach) pain, you may have pregnancy-induced hypertension (PIH). PIH (formerly called toxemia of pregnancy) refers to the development of hypertension, albuminuria (protein in the urine), or edema during the latter stage of pregnancy, usually between the twentieth week of pregnancy and the end of the first week postpartum. It may occur with or without convulsive seizures and coma. *Pre-eclampsia* (PIH without seizures or coma) develops in 5 percent of pregnant women. If left untreated, eclampsia (PIH with seizures or coma) usually ensues. You might feel fine; in fact, you may actually feel *more* energetic because of your elevated blood pressure, but this condition can be life-threatening.

If your blood pressure was elevated before you became pregnant or if you have a family history of hypertension, you may want to learn how to monitor your blood pressure at home. Ask your caregiver to recommend a monitoring device, many of which are now available in pharmacies and health food stores.

*Nutrition and Supplements*

PIH develops most often during the last three months of pregnancy. Food choices appear to play a role. Elevated blood levels of polyunsaturated fats, for example, have been noted in some women with PIH, and increasing the amount of linoleic acid (found in safflower oil, fish oils, and evening primrose oil) in the diet appears to help prevent or slow the development of PIH. If you have high blood pressure or a family history of high blood pressure, try eating more foods rich in linoleic acid (a fatty acid), such as fresh fish or fish oil supplements.

A Canadian study, reported in the September 1991 issue of the *Canadian Medical Association Journal,* found that women who ate fish and sea-mammal meat at least three times a week had lower average diastolic blood pressure levels during the last weeks of pregnancy.

Potassium-rich foods—such as bananas, orange juice, or lightly cooked organically grown potato peels—may also help regulate your blood pressure. Raw beets may also help. Try drinking raw beet root juice daily or adding beet roots to your salad. A fruit drink blended with *spirulina* (an alga) also helps lower high blood pressure levels. Spirulina is now available in capsules or powders. Adding young dandelion leaves (an excellent source of calcium and potassium) to salads will help take the strain off your kidneys by reducing edema. You can also drink a cup of dandelion tea twice daily.

Several studies suggest that PIH can be reduced with calcium and magnesium supplements. One study reported in the June 1990 issue of the *American Journal of Clinical Nutrition* that 19 women with PIH had low levels of magnesium and calcium during their thirty-fifth to forty-second weeks of pregnancy.

To prevent PIH, we recommend at least 1,200 milligrams of calcium and 320 milligrams of magnesium daily. Ask your caregiver about the possible benefit of increasing your daily intake of protein and vitamin $B_6$ (brewer's yeast is a good source) to prevent PIH.

## Edema

The technical term for tissue swelling is *edema,* which is usually caused by an increase in fluid volume. Hot weather, prolonged standing, or fatigue can make it worse. Tissue swelling is referred to as *pitting edema* when an indentation mark remains after finger pressure is applied. If you notice pitting edema in your legs or hands, you may also have PIH. Discuss any noticeable symptoms with your caregiver.

One way to reduce swelling in your feet is to avoid standing for long periods of time, especially in hot weather. At work, if possible, try to keep your feet elevated as often as possible. Women who must stand (nurses, for example), should try sleeping with their feet elevated on soft pillows.

| | |
|---|---|
| ***Ayurvedic Medicine*** | A helpful Ayurvedic therapy for edema is to boil four parts water with one part barley juice, strain the mixture, and drink it as a tea. Swelling can also be reduced by applying a mixture of turmeric (two parts) and salt (one part) to your feet and ankles. Ask your caregiver about taking 200 milligrams of the Indian herb pararnava guggulu twice a day after lunch and dinner. |
| ***Biofeedback*** | Simple biofeedback-assisted relaxation exercises that you can do at home can reduce swelling in your feet and ankles. One simple exercise can be done sitting or lying down: visualize the temperature of your toes increasing—this can reduce swelling for some women. |
| ***Botanical Medicine*** | Ask your caregiver about using hot ginger root compresses to reduce swelling in painful joints. The easiest method of preparing them is to fold fresh crushed ginger into hot towels and apply as a compress to an affected joint. Also, ask about taking dandelion or golden rod supplements to lower your blood pressure and reduce edema. |
| ***Homeopathy*** | Ask your homeopath about taking belladonna, aconite, ferrum phosphate, sulfur, or Natrum muriaticum to relieve edema. |
| ***Hydrotherapy*** | Immersing your feet in alternating hot and cold baths for thirty minutes at a time or applying damp towels to your feet will reduce swelling by accelerating the drainage of lymph (a clear fluid that removes the waste products of inflammation) and flow of fresh blood to the affected area. Alternatively, you can wrap ice cubes in a towel and use it to massage sore areas if the swelling persists. |
| ***Massage*** | Massage helps reverse leg swelling by opening drainage (lymphatic) channels. While reclining in a comfortable position, have your partner massage you from your toes towards your waist. Don't allow anyone to massage your heel, ankle bones, or Achilles tendon, because they are connected to nerve meridians in the uterus, and massage may stimulate contractions. Once you're in labor, however, massaging these areas is safe and can help relieve pain. |
| ***Nutrition and Supplements*** | Reducing your consumption of sodium-rich foods, commercial soft drinks, and refined sugars may reduce swelling. Raspberry leaf tea may also be beneficial. Drinking at least eight glasses of filtered water |

daily and dandelion tea will help flush out excess fluids from your tissues. Be sure to avoid an excessive intake of caffeinated beverages or undiluted fruit juices, which contain too much sugar.

Several vitamin and mineral supplements—including vitamins A, B, and C—have been used to help reduce edema. Bromelain supplements (made from pineapple) taken on an empty stomach are also beneficial.

*Osteopathy*

Cranial and osteopathic massage may help relieve pressure on the lower legs, enhance lymphatic flow, and reduce mild swelling.

# Insomnia

Hormonal changes, stress, the increasing activity of your baby, and ordinary discomforts during pregnancy can all keep you from sleeping. It's important for you to work with your caregiver to identify the cause of insomnia. Try nutrition, herbs, homeopathy, traditional Chinese medicine, Ayurvedic medicine, and behavior modification for relief. And remember: You need your rest during this special time. Taking naps during the day may help rebalance your circadian rhythms and help you sleep at night.

*Acupuncture*

Acupuncture balances the energy meridians and is very relaxing. It has been used to prevent and relieve insomnia.

*Aromatic Baths*

Some women find that soaking in a bath to which scents such as lavender have been added helps them sleep. When there's no time for a bath, drench a washcloth in one of these scents and inhale. If you wake up during the night, spray a small amount of Joie de Lavender Mist on your pillow to help ease yourself back to dreamland.

Some women find it helps to massage their foreheads with two or three drops of the sleep-inducing lavender oil mixed with almond oil.

*Ayurvedic Medicine*

Rubbing essential oils of coconut, sesame, or mustard on your forehead and feet before going to bed may help you sleep better.

*Bach Flower Remedies*

Midwives often recommend adding a few drops of Bach Rescue Remedy to a cup of warm water and drinking it as a nighttime tea. The tea is a safe and natural beverage, and will induce a quiet night's sleep.

| | |
|---|---|
| *Biofeedback* | Insomnia is often caused by overstimulation of the autonomic nervous system and by muscle tension. The biofeedback and relaxation exercises recommended for edema (see above) will also help you fall asleep. |
| *Botanical Medicines* | Chamomile or lime blossom tea mixed with skullcap may help relieve insomnia. Valerian supplements have also been proven safe and effective for helping women fall asleep. Linden flower, passion flower, and hops supplements are also effective; oils or extracts of these herbs can be added to your bath before going to bed. |
| *Exercise* | Twenty minutes of aerobic exercise in the late afternoon or early evening may help you sleep better. Early evening is a good time for light exercises, such as walking. Don't exercise just before going to sleep, however, because this will raise your heart rate and keep you awake. |
| *Homeopathy* | If it's very difficult for you to fall asleep, ask your homeopath for advice. He or she may recommend one tablet of Passiflor 6X, Coffea Cruda 6X, or Nux Vomica 6X before going to bed and another if you wake up during the night. |
| *Hydrotherapy* | Taking a warm bath to which baking soda has been added before retiring helps increase skin circulation and soothes the nerves. Adding two drops of pine needle essence, oil of eucalyptus, or mustard powder to the bath water is also helpful. |

*Controlled Breathing Exercise*

Controlled breathing exercises, such as those used with yoga, may help you fall asleep more quickly. The following breathing exercise may also induce drowsiness:

1. Lie on your side with your eyes closed and slowly inhale. Imagine filling your lungs completely.

2. Exhale fully, drawing in your abdomen to expel as much air as possible.

3. Repeat this procedure two or three times, until you feel drowsy.

| | |
|---|---|
| *Nutrition and Supplements* | Alcohol and caffeine can cause insomnia. Try avoiding them or limit your intake if you find it difficult to sleep. Avoiding cow's milk also helps some women sleep better. A protein-rich snack, such as yogurt, or taking one gram of vitamin $B_3$ at bedtime may help induce drowsiness. |
| *Progressive Relaxation* | Progressive relaxation exercises, in which you contract and relax neck and facial muscles in succession, also may help you fall asleep. Contract your facial muscles forcefully for one to two seconds, then relax them completely. If you repeat the procedure for all your facial and neck muscles, you will induce a deep state of relaxation sleepiness. |
| | You may also find it helpful to sleep with your legs raised slightly on pillows. Some women find this induces sleep. Be sure to empty your bladder when you feel the urge, because sleeping is much easier when your bladder is empty. |
| *Visualization* | Imagine yourself relaxing in a peaceful environment. For example, visualize yourself relaxing at the seashore, in the mountains, or in another peaceful environment. The important thing is that you set five to ten minutes aside each night before bedtime for this relaxation technique. |
| *Vitamin and Mineral Therapies* | Calcium, copper, iron, magnesium, phosphorous, and zinc deficiencies can cause irritability and nervousness, which interfere with sleeping. Ask your caregiver about increasing your daily intake of these nutrients or taking them as supplements. |

*Chapter* 7

# The Sixth Month

YOU'RE NOW ENTERING YOUR SIXTH MONTH of pregnancy. By the end of the month, your baby will be approximately thirteen to fifteen inches long and weigh about almost one and a quarter pounds. Baby's head is still by far the largest part of the body. You've probably already felt the baby moving inside you. You may find it slightly more difficult to move about now because of the increased size of your lower abdomen.

During this month, your baby's nails and hair will be growing. Baby will also start to develop fat and *vernix,* the oily substance that protects the skin against the effects of amniotic fluid. The nostrils will open, and the muscles involved with breathing will begin to contract. By now, the brainwave patterns are usually similar to those seen after birth. They are believed to originate from the more highly evolved part of the brain, the prefrontal cortex. It is believed that these waves reflect your baby's first attempts to hear and see.

## THE SIXTH-MONTH CHECKUP

During this month's checkup, your caregiver will continue to monitor your weight, blood pressure, blood, and urine, as well as the height of the fundus, the size and position of your uterus, and your baby's heartbeat. You will also be checked for signs of edema and asked about other symptoms of complications. If you haven't already enrolled in childbirth classes, ask your caregiver to recommend one. This is normally a quiet and comfortable month for women, but be sure to discuss holistic remedies for any new symptoms you might be experiencing, such as leg cramps, backaches, increased heart rate, hemorrhoids, toxemia, or rectal bleeding.

## HOLISTIC CHILDBIRTH CLASSES

Now is the time to start taking childbirth classes, if you haven't done so already. These classes will help you understand all your options for giving birth, including *where* and *how* you want to deliver your baby. Once you've checked into a hospital, it may be too late to change your mind.

The information offered in prenatal courses will answer many of your questions, especially those concerning exercise and nutrition, as well as relaxation and breathing exercises for labor and delivery. Childbirth classes also offer you an opportunity to discuss the safest and least invasive birthing options with other mothers as well as childbirth educators and midwives. Numerous studies have shown that these classes help reduce a mother's anxiety and increase her confidence and ability to relax during labor and delivery.

Look for courses run by hospitals, public health organizations, private instructors, holistic caregivers, and former mothers. "Early bird" prenatal classes may be available. These are taken in the first or second trimester and cover nutrition, exercise, fetal development, hygiene, sexuality, and dreams and fantasies. There are also late classes, usually for women in the seventh or eighth month of pregnancy, which focus on labor, delivery, and postpartum care for mother and baby.

### Grantly Dick-Read Classes

Grantly Dick-Read, M.D., an English obstetrician, believed that a pregnant woman's fear of childbirth disturbs nerve–muscle interactions during labor and produces tension, which is perceived as pain. To counter this, he developed childbirth classes in which pregnant women are coached to relax and breathe appropriately during labor contractions. Dick-Read classes also stress the importance of choosing a birth attendant you trust and are comfortable with. They also strongly recommend that the father attend classes and serve as a coach in the labor and delivery room. Women are usually advised to begin the program in the fourth month of pregnancy. Classes are conducted by instructors certified in the *Gamper method,* named for Margaret Gamper, the nurse who inspired Dr. Dick-Read. Addresses and phone numbers of childbirth programs appear in Appendix C.

## Psychopro-phylaxis

Psychoprophylaxis was developed in Russia in the 1940s. Like the Dick-Read program, psychoprophylaxis is based on the belief that pain is a learned reflex and that women can be re-educated to avoid focusing on pain during labor. Mothers are also taught anatomy, breathing techniques, relaxation, pushing methods, and positions to use during labor. In the United States, psychoprophylaxis has been combined with the Lamaze method (see below).

## ASPO/Lamaze

The Lamaze technique, developed by Frederick Lamaze, a French obstetrician, is a modified method of psychoprophylaxis. Lamaze classes teach mothers to replace pain and fear with joyful expectation and to view labor contractions as sensations instead of birth pains. The American Society for Psychoprophylaxis in Obstetrics (ASPO/Lamaze) is a nonprofit society that was founded in 1960. ASPO/Lamaze–trained instructors teach breathing, relaxation, and delivery exercises, such as pant-blow breathing, to help women control their pushing urges during labor. Members of ASPO/Lamaze include childbirth educators, nurses, nurse-midwives, and physicians, as well as consumers who support Lamaze childbirth methods.

ASPO/Lamaze has an internationally recognized certification program for childbirth educators and has licensed more than 10,000 educators. Approximately 150,000 Lamaze classes are taught each year and are attended by more than 2 million parents. According to ASPO/Lamaze statistics, one fourth of American women who have given birth attended classes taught by ASPO-certified Childbirth Educators (ACCEs).

## The Bradley Method

Developed by an American obstetrician, the Bradley method combines Lamaze and Dick-Read methods. Women are trained in relaxation exercises for labor, and the role of the father or partner as labor coach is strongly emphasized. Mothers learn to use slower, lower diaphragm breathing exercises during labor. Instead of helping women focus on external distractions to overcome their perception of pain, the Bradley method helps women understand and concentrate on what's happening inside their bodies. Pain relievers and medication are recommended only for complications and cesarean deliveries, and 94 percent of Bradley-trained mothers give birth without them. "Early bird" Bradley classes are offered in most cities, as are classes that continue into the postpartum period, although they aren't mandatory. A typical Bradley course lasts twelve weeks, beginning in the fifth or sixth month.

## Other Classes

Classes are also offered privately by childbirth educators certified by the International Childbirth Education Association. These educators support family-centered maternity care and a minimum of medical intervention. Some hospitals also provide childbirth classes, as do

## ESPECIALLY *for* FATHERS

CHILDBIRTH CLASSES are an excellent way to become a primary support person during pregnancy and birth. The support person can be someone other than the father, of course. Most classes include information on the physical process of pregnancy, labor, and delivery and teach couples how to use breathing and relaxation techniques during labor. The support person's role during labor and birth is emphasized, and teamwork between you and your partner is encouraged. You're also urged to practice these skills together in advance at home.

If you have any questions, childbirth classes are a good place to have them answered. The goal of these classes is to make you and your partner as informed and comfortable as possible. Talk with your partner about what she expects of you and how involved you want to be during labor and delivery.

health maintenance organizations (HMOs) and other health care providers. Some cities also provide pregnancy and childbirth education in local high schools or junior colleges.

## *H*OLISTIC APPROACHES TO COMMON SIXTH-MONTH CONCERNS

**Leg Cramps**

With the changes in your body and so much on your mind, you probably have enough trouble sleeping without having to suffer from leg cramps. Mildly painful spasms, which usually occur at night, are common during the second and third trimesters. Mild legs cramps normally last only a few minutes. They are usually caused by the additional weight you're carrying, circulatory changes, or a calcium deficiency. You can prevent cramps by exercising regularly (see Chapter 4) and taking calcium and magnesium supplements. Also, try wearing shoes with good arch supports, since your increased weight may be flattening the arch of your foot. If the pain persists, try acupuncture or acupressure, both of which are effective in relieving symptoms, or ask your caregiver about vitamin E supplements, which reduce pain for some women.

*Massage*

Often you can relieve a leg cramp with self-massage. As soon as you notice a cramp, massage and stretch your leg muscles by extending your heel and bringing your toes toward you, or try the following exercise to get rid of a spasm:

1. Stand two feet away from a wall, with the cramping leg farther away from the wall than the other leg. Put your hands against the wall, then bend your front knee and lean forward.

2. Keeping your back knee straight, move your rear foot as far back as you can without lifting your heel.

3. Hold this pose for a few seconds, dropping your weight onto your back heel.

4. Relax, change legs, and repeat this exercise several times.

*Physical Activity*

You can usually relieve a mild cramp by gently massaging your leg muscles and then gently stretching them. Try the following exercise after the massage:

1. Lie on your left side, with your shoulders, hips, and knees in a straight line.

2. Place your right hand on the floor in front of your chest and support your head with your left hand.

3. Relax and inhale. Then exhale while slowly raising your right leg as high as you can, keeping your foot flexed (toes pointing toward your belly) and your inner ankle facing directly down. Your leg can be either straight or bent at the knee, whichever is more comfortable.

4. Inhale while slowly lowering your leg.

5. Repeat ten times on each side.

## Backaches

The weight of your growing baby puts more pressure on the natural curve of your spine and can cause lower back pain. The extra weight is borne mainly by your lower back but is transferred through the lower vertebrae (bones) of the spine to your hips, legs, and feet.

The way you sit, sleep, and walk will affect the amount of stress on your back. Try sleeping on a firm mattress and sitting upright with your back well supported and both feet flat on the floor. Always wear shoes with good arch support, and keep your head erect, shoulders back, and buttocks tucked in when you walk.

If you don't think these posture tips are important, try this experiment at home. Hold a mop or broom upright, with the business end up in the air. Notice how little effort this takes, as long as the broom remains perfectly upright. Now allow the mop or broom to lean slightly to one side and try to hold it in that position. Feel how much tighter your grip becomes? Feel how your arm muscles tense up? Feel your whole arm start trembling? That's how much harder your back muscles must work when you slouch or overarch your back.

Your body really wants to be efficient. Poor posture makes the muscles work so much harder—no wonder they get tired!

Poor posture can lead to the compression of the *intervertebral disks,* which lie between the vertebrae of the spine and act as vertical "shock absorbers." It can also put pressure on the *spinal nerves,* which run through little "windows" created by the interlocking facets on adjacent vertebrae. This pressure causes an extremely painful condition. Good posture, on the other hand, helps maintain adequate spaces between the vertebrae.

| | |
|---|---|
| *Botanical Medicine* | Your caregiver or herbalist should help you identify the precise cause of your back pain. If your pain is related to excessive physical strain or rheumatic (inflammatory) problems, your caregiver may recommend drinking meadowsweet tea three times a day. Rubbing your back with a tincture of lobelia may also relieve pain. |
| *Physical Activity* | An easy way to relieve back pain is to gently massage your back with two tennis balls wrapped in a towel or sock. Lie down on a firm surface and place the balls about one inch apart underneath the tightest parts of your back muscles. Breathe deeply for one minute. Then move so that the balls roll to another tight or painful area. Continue to breathe deeply for another minute. Another exercise involves firmly bringing your knees into your chest several times. Repeat this two or three times daily to prevent and relieve back pain. |
| *Acupuncture* | Acupuncture is also effective for relieving back pain. It is wonderfully relaxing—it can even be used during labor. Be sure that you see a practitioner who specializes in treating pregnant women. |
| *Aromatherapy* | For upper back pain and fatigue, try inhaling an infusion of lavender, marjoram, rosemary, or sage. For prolonged pain, try an infusion of black pepper, ginger, or birch. |
| *Ayurvedic Medicine* | Ask an Ayurvedic physician about *Kairhore guggulu* (an Indian herb) supplements or *dashamoola basti* tea. Massaging painful parts of the back with mahanarayan oil may also relieve symptoms. |
| *Biofeedback* | Ask your caregiver to show you how to use biofeedback to voluntarily relax your back muscles. Once you've learned the technique, you can use it at home whenever your muscles become fatigued or tense. |
| *Chiropractic* | Chiropractic is a safe and easy way of relieving back pain during pregnancy and labor. In *Everybody's Guide to Chiropractic Health Care*, Nathaniel Altman describes an American study in which 82 percent of 400 pregnant women "experienced less pain during labor" after they had a chiropractic alignment. |

| | |
|---|---|
| ***Hydrotherapy*** | Applying hot, moist compresses made with water and hot apple cider vinegar to the lower back may be helpful. Another beneficial treatment is the alternating of hot and cold showers on painful areas. |

Ice is one of the most effective methods for treating back pain, especially when there is swelling, heat, or redness in the painful area. Ice causes the narrowing of blood vessels leading to the painful area, reducing the amount of fluid and inflammation-causing substances to that area. It is particularly effective when the pain first develops. A standard treatment is to apply ice for ten minutes, heat for five minutes, and continue alternating them as often as needed throughout the day. If swelling and pain continue, discuss the problem with your caregiver.

***Massage***

Bend your knees slightly, keeping your upper back straight and your shoulders relaxed. Raise your arms gently above your head. Have your partner gently massage your lower back, stroking firmly downward, around your hips, and along your legs.

***Qigong***

Tai chi and qigong will help you to learn to stand and walk correctly by evenly distributing your weight on your feet, with your feet facing forward and parallel to each other. You'll notice that turning your feet out, for example, puts a strain on your lower back and knee joints. When you learn to loosen your knees and position your pelvis correctly—by lengthening your lower back and tucking your tailbone under—you'll be amazed how few backaches develop.

Qigong exercises help you bring your body into alignment so that your abdomen is well supported. Try not to hollow or arch your lower back, because this will throw your belly forward, thereby straining muscles in your abdomen and in the lower part of your spine. When sitting, avoid crossing your legs and be sure to straighten your spine by lengthening your lower back. When lifting objects or children, squat down with your feet flat on the floor and aligned with your shoulders rather than bending forward. Stand up slowly, aligning your spine to avoid straining your back.

***Yoga***

Several of the towel and yoga exercises described in Chapter 4 will help you gently stretch your back, increase your circulation, strengthen your pelvic muscles, and relieve lower-back pain and bloating.

The following exercise will gently stretch your back and relieve temporary pains. As you do this exercise, try not to hold your breath or inhale forcefully.

1.  Sit in a kneeling position with your buttocks resting on your heels, keeping your head, neck, and trunk straight.

2.  Relax your arms and rest your hands on the floor, your palms facing upward and fingers pointing behind you.

3.  Exhaling, slowly bend forward from your hips until your stomach and chest rest lightly on your thighs.

| | |
|---|---|
| **Abdominal Pain** | During pregnancy, you may feel a variety of abdominal pains which are usually associated with muscular changes or the growth of your uterus. They are rarely serious. Sometimes they occur when your uterus turns slightly to one side or the other—usually to the right. Such twisting produces a pulling sensation, usually in the lower right side of the abdomen. You'll notice them when you get up quickly or turn sharply from one side to the other. The baby can also cause abdominal pain by kicking. Some babies just keep bumping and kicking the same spot over and over, causing discomfort. It's important, however, to inform your caregiver of any severe pains that do not go away, as they may require treatment. |
| *Massage* | Massaging your abdominal muscles every day during pregnancy helps keep them supple and prepares them for labor and delivery. You can use twelve ounces of natural wheat germ or almond oil combined with an ounce of lavender or apricot kernel extract. Apply the oil to your belly and abdomen with smooth circular strokes, working in a clockwise direction. Continue to oil and massage your hips and thighs and the rest of your body, too. |
| *Yoga (***Reclining Cobblers** *Pose, with Chest Support)* | The next two yoga poses, recommended by Dr. Mary Schatz in her book, *Back Care Basics: A Doctor's Gentle Yoga Program for Back and Neck Pain Relief,* will help relax abdominal cramps by gently exercising your pelvis and inner thighs. Be sure to do the poses very slowly so that you don't distend your stomach muscles or strain your uterine muscles. |

1. Get a blanket and a towel. Fold the blanket several times and roll the towel. Sit on the floor, facing a wall, with the blanket behind you, touching your buttocks. Keep the towel within reach.

2. Slowly fold your legs in toward your body so that the soles of your feet are touching each other and your toes are pressing against the wall.

3. Using your arms for support, roll your spine down onto the blanket. Support your head and neck comfortably with the rolled towel. Then spread your arms out to either side with your palms facing up.

4. If your inner thighs feel overstretched, support each knee with folded blankets or move your buttocks farther away from the wall, so that there's more distance between your feet and buttocks. Hold the pose for several breaths.

## Urinary Incontinence

In the second and third trimesters, some women start to leak small amounts of urine, usually when they laugh, cough, or sneeze. This incontinence results from the mounting pressure of your growing uterus against your bladder. Kegel exercises, which are useful for firming up pelvic muscles for delivery and postpartum recovery, usually help control incontinence. If your secretions are clear, pinkish, or greenish-yellow, there is a slight chance that you're leaking amniotic fluid. You should report this to your caregiver immediately.

### Kegel Exercises

Kegel exercises, which strengthen the perineal muscles, will also strengthen the sphincters ("valves") that control the flow of urine from the bladder and help relieve incontinence.

1. Pretend that your vagina is an elevator shaft with five floors and a basement. Pretend that the level at which your perineal muscles are normally at rest is the first floor.

2. Tighten slowly up to the second "floor" of the vagina. Tighten again slowly up to the third floor, then the fourth, and finally the fifth (top) floor.

3. Hold your muscles here for ten seconds, then very slowly release down to the fourth floor and hold for five seconds, to the third floor, and hold for 10 seconds, the second floor and hold, and finally the first floor and hold.

4.  Gently push your muscles downward to the "basement."

5.  Now pull your muscles back up to the first floor.

## Varicose Veins

As noted earlier, your blood volume increases during pregnancy to support the growth of your baby and your supporting body tissues. The extra fluid in the lower part of your body can cause the veins in your legs, vulva, and rectum to become swollen, or *varicose.* These varicosities can be unsightly, painful, and itchy. Vulval varicosities usually disappear after childbirth. Varicose veins in your legs, however, may not disappear. Holistic medicine focuses on preventing varicose veins through a high-fiber diet, gradual weight gain, exercise, massage, acupuncture, and homeopathic or botanical medicines approved by your caregiver.

### *Botanical Medicine*

For varicose veins in the legs, botanicals such as horse chestnut, nettle, yarrow, St. John's Wort, and shepherd's purse, applied externally, help to improve blood flow. Ask your caregiver or herbalist for a lotion containing these substances. An ointment of comfrey, yellow dock root, plantain, or yarrow may also help ease the pain of varicose veins. In addition, witch hazel, applied on a lint compress to affected areas, will ease symptoms, as will lemon juice or apple cider vinegar, although these may sting a little.

For varicose veins in the vulva, apply grated raw potato and ice compresses to your perineum. Also, try taking a cold shower and directing the water between your legs. Horse chestnut ointments applied locally may also be helpful.

### *Physical Activity*

Brisk walking, jogging, and swimming are recommended by the American College of Obstetricians and Gynecologists (ACOG) as ideal (see Chapter 4) for increasing blood circulation and preventing varicose veins.

An easy way to prevent varicose veins in your legs and feet is to always sit or sleep with your feet elevated. Avoid prolonged standing; if you have to stand for long periods of time, rest one foot on a low box or stool. If you're in a grocery line, for example, rest your foot on the lower rack of the grocery cart. When working in the kitchen, open a cabinet door and rest your foot on the lower shelf.

Try not to sit in one position for more than half an hour when you're eating or working. Keep a small box, footstool, or thick telephone book nearby and rest one or both feet on it. Don't sit with your legs crossed, as that prevents blood from flowing freely.

*Homeopathy*

For painful varicose veins, ask your homeopath about taking Hamamelis 6X, which is usually taken three times daily up to a week. Calcarea fluorica 6X is excellent for strengthening elastic tissue and preventing varicose veins from developing again. For external application, midwives often recommend adding one tablespoon of arnica tincture to a liter of cold water and applying it twice daily to affected areas, using a saturated washcloth.

*Hydrotherapy*

Herbal baths relieve both varicose veins and hemorrhoids effectively. Just add four ounces of witch hazel and two ounces of comfrey root to four pints of water and let it sit for eight hours. Then strain the residue and pour into a hot bath. Sit in the solution for fifteen minutes twice daily.

*Nutrition and Supplements*

Raw garlic, onions, and parsley increase the elasticity of veins and prevent constipation, which often leads to varicose veins in the rectum. Sunflower seeds and wheat germ, both rich in vitamin E, have also been demonstrated to prevent varicose veins. A daily vitamin E supplement of 600 international units is usually recommended to help repair broken capillaries. Rutin supplements also reduce varicose veins, although they should not be taken until the fourth month of pregnancy. Buckwheat, for example, is a good source of rutin. Increasing your intake of vitamin C-rich foods, such as citrus fruits or raw beets, will also prevent or relieve the symptoms of varicose veins.

Ask your caregiver about the usefulness of vitamins $B_1$, C, and E supplements in preventing varicose veins.

## Chapter 8

# The Seventh Month

Y OUR THIRD TRIMESTER HAS ARRIVED!

By the beginning of the twenty-fifth week, your baby will be almost sixteen inches long and weigh two to two-and-a-half pounds. By the end of this month, your baby's eyes will be completely formed and the taste buds will be working. If your baby were born at the end of twenty-eight weeks, it would have a good chance of surviving.

The third trimester is a time of great physical and emotional change. Your body is making its final adaptations to give birth, and this often produces new discomforts, such as lower abdominal pain, overheating, and bladder discomfort. By the end of this month, your baby's movements may become very strong, noticeable, and varied. Don't be concerned if you feel the movements a bit earlier or later than this month. In some pregnancies, the movements are very weak; in others, they are very strong. You may feel a rhythmic tapping inside your abdomen, which indicates baby hiccups. These are normal contractions of your baby's diaphragm as your child makes his or her first attempts at breathing.

You'll need to begin to modify your diet and exercise program to prepare for labor and childbirth. You'll also have to learn how to deal with fluctuating emotions. This chapter explains how to modify your food plan and exercise program, and also how to deal with common sexual and emotional changes during the third trimester. You may also have questions about using pain relievers during labor. In this chapter, we provide holistic guidelines that will make sure that you give yourself and your baby the best chance for a successful natural childbirth. You should be attending childbirth classes now in preparation for labor and delivery. Along with talking regularly with your caregiver, you'll find the classes invaluable for preparing you for the event.

## THE SEVENTH-MONTH CHECKUP

By now, you should have already arranged with your caregiver how and where you want to deliver your baby. If you haven't, you should resolve any last-minute concerns about your Birth Plan during this month's checkup. Usually by the third trimester, women feel less ambivalent about their ability to go through childbirth. If you still have lingering doubts, you should talk about these as well.

The added weight and movement of your baby may cause new discomforts this month, such as lower abdominal pain, overheating, baby kicks, bladder discomfort, and fatigue. Your caregiver should be able to recommend holistic remedies for these discomforts.

Be sure to discuss anything unusual you may have noticed about your baby's movement. If you've had a baby before, it's easier to recognize normal movement. Usually, you're able to feel your baby moving earlier in your second pregnancy than in your first.

## COMMON SEVENTH-MONTH CONCERNS

### Nutrition during the Third Trimester

You should discuss with your caregiver adding more protein to your diet. Research has shown that inadequate protein intake in expectant mothers, along with low caloric intake, can result in babies being smaller than normal at birth. You should consume at least 60 to 75 grams of protein daily; some nutritionists recommend 100 grams. Mothers who experience nausea and vomiting may need more and should consume at least four servings of protein each day. You can fulfill your protein requirements by eating high-protein snacks such as nuts and seeds, soy-based foods, yogurt, cheese, or wheat germ.

Also, make sure you're still getting enough iron and calcium. If you're not taking supplements already, discuss them with your caregiver. To increase your calcium intake, try low-fat milk or milk products, tofu, or fish with edible bones, such as salmon or sardines.

## DIETARY GUIDELINES FOR THE THIRD TRIMESTER

You can meet the RDAs for essential vitamins and minerals during the third trimester of your pregnancy by following these guidelines:

1. Consume at least five daily servings of fresh fruits and vegetables, especially orange or dark green vegetables and citrus fruits.

2. Consume at least six servings of whole-grain breads and cereals each day.

3. Limit dietary fat intake to less than 30 percent of total calories, saturated fat to less than 10 percent of calories, and cholesterol to less than 300 milligrams per day.

4. Consume between 25 and 35 grams of fiber each day.

5. Consume at least three to four calcium-rich foods daily, including nonfat or low-fat milk.

6. If you cannot get the amount of iron you need from foods, take a daily supplement of thirty milligrams of ferrous iron. To enhance iron absorption, take the supplement between meals with a vitamin C-rich fruit juice, such as orange juice.

7. Discuss your total caloric needs with your caregiver. Select less nutritious foods only after all your other nutritional needs for the day have been met, and limit your sugar intake to less than 10 percent of calories. Include a moderate-dose vitamin–mineral supplement if your calorie intake drops below 2,000 calories. The supplement should include fluoride if local drinking water is not fluoridated.

8. Drink at least eight 8-ounce glasses of fluids, especially water, each day.

9. Balance your caloric intake with exercise to keep from gaining weight too rapidly.

10. Avoid all alcoholic beverages until after the baby is born and then, if you must, drink only in moderation.

11. Limit salt intake.

12. Divide your meals into several small meals and snacks rather than just a few large meals if indigestion is still a problem.

## Physical Activity during the Third Trimester

During the third trimester, you'll need to modify your exercise routine to accommodate several physical changes. Your center of gravity shifts during the last trimester because of your increased weight. Avoid any exercise or sports that might cause you to lose your balance. Walking and swimming are ideal. ACOG provides the following guidelines for women during the third trimester:

1. Avoid putting pressure on your abdomen and pelvis. As the fetus grows, your internal organs are pushed closer to your diaphragm and your rib cage expands laterally to maintain your breathing capacity. Avoid exercises, such as rowing, that put pressure on your abdomen.

2. Avoid exercising on your back. ACOG advises pregnant women not to exercise while lying on their backs after the fourth month of pregnancy, because the fetus may be large enough to interfere with blood flow through major blood vessels. For this reason, pregnant women are advised not to do traditional sit-ups or abdominal crunches.

3. Avoid high-intensity exercises. As your uterus increases in size, your lung space is reduced. Meanwhile, your baby needs more oxygen for aerobic activity. Switch from high-impact to low-impact aerobic activity to avoid becoming short of breath.

4. Strengthen your spinal muscles. Your additional weight puts additional stress on your lower back. You can counteract this by performing some of the gentle, low-impact yoga exercises described in Chapter 4 to strengthen your gluteal muscles and stretch your spinal muscles.

Remember: regular exercise helps condition you for labor and birth, helps control your weight gain, enhances your appearance, and makes you feel good about yourself. So whatever you do, don't stop exercising unless told to do so by your caregiver. If you can't motivate yourself to follow this exercise program at home, join an exercise class. Look for classes taught by midwives or experienced mothers, which focus on training the lower body muscles for labor and delivery.

## Emotional Changes during the Third Trimester

The third trimester is a time of change in many aspects of your life, not the least of which is sexual. Some women develop a heightened zest for sex during the last trimester. Other women lose their desire for sex or have difficulty becoming aroused. These changes are perfectly normal.

The important thing is to recognize that your sexual feelings (and those of your partner) may be more erratic than erotic. You may feel sexy one day and not the next. Mutual understanding and open communication are really important at this time in your lives.

Many changes caused by pregnancy increase the risk of problems in the relationship of the parents. However, that risk is much lower if couples talk about their concerns regularly. Communication, affection, and romance are important for your relationship and for your baby's well-being. If you notice that you're having sexual or communication problems, you're better off discussing these problems immediately, rather than waiting until after your baby is born. Effective communication requires both talking and listening. If you feel tired or overstressed, arrange to talk at a more convenient time. You and your partner will need to make a special effort to be empathetic to each other's feelings. If you find that you and your partner cannot resolve troubling issues on your own, it's a good idea to seek professional counseling.

### *Dreams*

Don't be surprised if you daydream or wake up in the middle of the night in the midst of a wild fantasy. Mothers often report dreaming about feeling trapped, not being able to protect their baby, losing things, missing a doctor's appointment, being unprepared for the baby when it arrives, gaining too much weight, and eating or drinking the wrong thing.

You'll find that dreams are a treasure trove of wisdom. They often help you sort out worries and fears in a nonthreatening way. They also can be seen as little messages from your subconscious about what you can do to make your pregnancy more enjoyable. It's a good idea to record your dreams on paper or on tape, even if you can remember only an image or a feeling. If you have trouble remembering your dreams, tell yourself before going to sleep that you want to remember your dream. Chances are, you will. Dating each dream and giving it a title will help you connect it with themes and events in your conscious life.

Be especially attentive to the emotions in your dreams. Try to listen to what your dreams are telling you about your feelings and deal with them. Some women find it helpful to program their dreams, by mentally affirming as they're about to fall asleep that they're going to dream about creative, intuitive solutions for their problems or worries.

# Especially *for* Fathers

DURING THE LAST THREE MONTHS OF PREGNANCY, your partner will go through new physical and emotional changes. She may be more uncomfortable because of her weight gain, she may feel more tired, and her breasts and abdomen may be very sore. These and other changes will effect her mood and her sexual desire. She may also crave more intimacy and feel more dependent on you. If you're taking childbirth classes together, you're probably already aware of the little (and big) things you can do to provide comfort and support. If you're not taking classes, reading this chapter will give you more suggestions.

During the last trimester of pregnancy, some women become fearful that they don't have enough love to share with both their baby and their partner. That's why it's especially important that you give her as much support and reassurance as you can during the final weeks.

Romance and sex are still very important. Invite your partner to take an unplanned evening walk, set aside time for cuddling and kissing, or enjoy a candle-lit dinner. Making a special effort to add one of these to each day of the week will make a world of difference for your relationship.

You could also work together to prepare the baby's room. Buying baby furniture and baby clothes together gets you both out of the house, gives her some exercise, and increases your shared anticipation of the big day.

You and your partner probably have already decided where and how the baby will be delivered and under what circumstances different pain relievers will be administered. You should familiarize yourself with all the pain relievers discussed in this chapter and help your partner decide which, if any, she's most comfortable with. You, your partner, and your caregiver are a team, and you all need to be on the same page. The more your partner feels that you understand her concerns, the more relaxed and confident she'll be during labor and childbirth.

***Nesting***

You'll spend a good deal of time in the final months of pregnancy creating a loving and stimulating environment for your baby—this is called the *nesting instinct*. Nesting is a good example of how to use your intuition to prepare for a pleasurable, relaxed, childbirth (see Box).

---

### PREPARING YOUR BABY'S ROOM

Here are some suggestions for creating a safe and stimulating environment for your baby:

▷ *Floor.* Washable floor rugs are best, because they provide noise control, warmth, and cushioning for falls. Pick an easily washable, nonflammable carpet made of polypropylene or cotton; nylon, orlon, wool and silk carpets can emit highly toxic fumes if burned. If you have hardwood floors, use a throw rug and place a nonslip rubber mat under it.

▷ *Painting floors, walls, etc.* Lead-based paint isn't sold anymore, but you should be concerned about the paint already on the walls in your home. If you believe there may be lead paint under your current paint—especially around window ledges—have it scraped off and repainted with semi-gloss paint, which is the easiest to wipe clean. Don't paint or strip paint while you're pregnant.

▷ *Crib.* Your baby furniture should be sturdy and made of unpainted natural woods with rounded corners. Don't use pillows, since the baby won't have much control over his or her head and could be easily smothered by them. Also, don't put stuffed animals with buttons or other decorations that baby can pull off and swallow in the crib. Crib bumpers should have at least six sets of straps or ties for the snuggest fit, but make sure the ties aren't more than six inches long.

▷ *Lights.* Place a small lamp on a bureau or shelf. This diffused lighting is more pleasing to the infant than bright overhead lights. A night-light will allow you to check on your baby without stumbling about in the dark. All lights should be out of the baby's reach.

▷ *Toys.* Be selective; buy only toys that stimulate your baby and develop his or her focusing abilities. A mobile over the crib or changing table should face the baby and have replaceable hanging elements to keep the baby from getting bored. Attach a shatterproof mirror to the crib slats—babies love human faces, including their own.

## Concerns about Work

A good job can supply friends, fulfillment, and money to do the things you want—all of which are key ingredients to happiness. Of course, it can also devour your time when you're pregnant and contribute additional stress. Whether you should work late into your pregnancy will

---

### H O W   L O N G   S H O U L D   I   W O R K ?

AMA now recommends that women whose jobs require them to remain on their feet more than four hours a day should quit by the twenty-fourth week; those who must stand for thirty minutes each hour should quit by the thirty-second week. If you're underweight and work, you risk gaining less weight during pregnancy and are at a greater risk of having a small baby—so you should quit or reduce your hours. Other recommendations of the AMA include the following:

▷ You can work safely until labor if your job is sedentary and not stressful. Don't work past the twentieth week if your job requires heavy lifting or pushing, climbing stairs, or bending below the waist. The AMA also recommends that you stop working after the twentieth week if your work shift changes, your appetite decreases, you're increasingly fatigued, or cannot sleep regularly. If this is not possible because you need your income, try to reduce your hours, and make a special effort to follow the therapies in this book for maintaining your appetite (eat six small meals instead of three large meals throughout the day), and for relieving fatigue, anemia, and insomnia.

▷ Get adequate rest and regular sleep. Rest and sleep regenerate your energy and are very important for your baby's biorhythms. If you plan to work until labor, it is absolutely essential that you sleep a minimum of eight hours in a restful state.

▷ Eat a healthy diet. Hectic lifestyles can lead to hectic eating styles, and inadequate nutrition during pregnancy can hamper your ability to handle stress as well as affect your baby's growth and development. Eat a minimum of three, preferably six small meals daily, take supplements, and start each day with a nutritious breakfast.

▷ Leave your work at the workplace. Don't take it home with you. Combat stress with any activity you find relaxing, such as sports, reading, going to the movies, socializing with friends, listening to music, or taking long walks during lunch.

▷ Wear support hose if your work involves long periods of standing. If you must stand for long periods of time, keep one foot on a low stool with your knee bent to take pressure off your back. If you work at a desk, keep your legs elevated on a stool or chair.

▷ Take frequent breaks and do stretching exercises, especially for your back and legs. Remember to empty your bladder every two hours.

depend on your family's economic needs, your employer's maternity leave policies, and, most importantly, your emotional needs and your caregiver's advice.

This would be a good time to review the specific details of your health insurance benefits and your employer's policies regarding flexible work schedules—such as part-time work, job sharing, or working from home.

***On-the-Job Stress Reduction Techniques***

If working helps take your mind off the discomforts of pregnancy, it shouldn't be harmful. If too much job-related stress leaves you feeling anxious or depressed, or causes headaches, backaches, or a loss of appetite, then try to reduce your hours. Reactions to stress—such as appetite loss, bingeing on the wrong foods, or sleeplessness—can take a toll on you and your baby. One way to avoid this is to practice the stress reduction exercises below:

1. Eye exercises. Close your eyes and roll your eyeballs upward. Take two deep breaths.

2. Roll-arounds. Roll your head in a circle several times and then reverse direction. Repeat several times, each time rolling more slowly and fully.

3. Lean-tos. Lean from side to side in your chair with your arms hanging until your hand is touching the floor with each lean.

4. Mini-mind visualizations. Close your eyes and visualize yourself in your favorite place—the mountains, in bed, etc. Stay there in your mind until your body feels it's there, too. If you have cold hands or feet, visualize yourself in a warm, friendly place.

## Pain Relievers

Every mother eagerly awaits the birth of her child, but very few look forward to the pain of labor that precedes it. This brings the following question to every mother's mind: Should I or shouldn't I take pain relievers?

Prudent use of any type of pain relief medication always requires weighing its risks against its benefits. In the case of pain relief drugs used during labor and delivery, the risks and benefits of each drug affect the health of you and your baby. Your caregiver may feel that the risk of your using pain relievers outweighs the benefits they offer. He or she may advise you against taking pain relief medication, for example, if your fetus does not appear strong enough to cope with the combined stress of labor and drugs. Your caregiver also may advise you not to take pain relievers if they might slow down your normal contractions. If your caregiver thinks the fetus is in trouble or that your uterus is not contracting, you may be advised not to take pain relief medication, and instead have your labor induced with Pitocin. Be sure to discuss with your caregiver the risks and benefits of taking any type of medication.

There are times, however, when medications are safe and necessary. ACOG guidelines recommend medication when:

▷ A mother is so agitated that her state of mind is hindering the progress of labor

▷ A precipitous (dangerously rapid) labor must be slowed down

▷ Outlet forceps (to ease the baby out once its head is visible at the vaginal outlet) are required

▷ Labor is long and complicated, since pain and stress can lead to chemical imbalances that can interfere with contractions, compromise blood flow to the uterus, and exhaust the mother, reducing her ability to push effectively

▷ The pain is more than the mother can tolerate or is interfering with her ability to dilate or push

## Holistic Guidelines for Using Pain Relievers

The holistic rule is to always select a pain relief drug that (1) has minimal side effects, (2) presents the least mind/body risk to you and your baby, and (3) can be administered late enough during labor to not affect your baby. General anesthesia is rarely used for cesarean deliveries, for example, because the fetus would have to be extracted within minutes after the drug is administered to the mother, before it has a chance to cross the placenta in significant amounts.

Minimizing the effect of drugs on the baby is important to prevent having a sluggish, unresponsive baby, possibly with breathing or sucking difficulties or an irregular heartbeat. Studies show that the fetus can handle a certain degree of depressed activity due to medication during labor or delivery. Certain drugs, however, can depress your baby's immune system.

A variety of *analgesics* (pain relievers), *anesthetics* (substances that produce loss of sensation), and tranquilizers may be given during labor and delivery. It's important to know the appropriate use of each. The decision to use specific drugs (if any) will depend on the stage of your labor, your past health history, and the preferences of you and your caregiver.

*Analgesics*

Meperidine is one of the most frequently used analgesic pain relievers. It's usually administered intravenously (injected slowly into an IV apparatus), or intramuscularly (one shot given in a large muscle group, usually the buttocks). It may be given every two to four hours, as needed. This drug does not usually interfere with contractions, although in large doses it may cause them to become less frequent or weaker. Like other analgesics, meperidine is not generally administered until labor is well established and false labor has been ruled out. It's usually discontinued three to four hours before delivery.

Some women find that meperidine relaxes them and makes them better able to cope with contractions. Others dislike the drowsy feeling it causes and find they are less able to cope with labor. Side effects may include (depending on individual sensitivity) nausea, vomiting, depression, and lowered blood pressure.

Meperidine's effect on your baby depends on the total dose and how close to delivery it is administered. If it is given too close to delivery, the baby may be sleepy and unable to suck. These effects are generally short-term and, if necessary, can be counteracted. Meperidine may also be given postpartum to relieve the pain of an episiotomy repair or cesarean delivery.

*Tranquilizers*

Promethazine and hydroxyzine are used to relax women who become nervous during labor. Like analgesics, tranquilizers are usually administered once labor is well established.

Some expectant mothers welcome the gentle drowsiness tranquilizers produce; others find that it interferes with their ability to control pushing. Smaller doses can be administered safely to relieve anxiety without impairing alertness. Larger doses often cause slurring of speech and dozing between contraction peaks, which make the use of holistic procedures more difficult. Although the risk of tranquilizers causing fetal distress or being dangerous for babies at risk for fetal distress is minimal, you and your caregiver should try non-drug relaxation techniques first before resorting to medication.

***Regional Nerve Blocks***

Regional anesthetics are used to completely numb the pelvic area during a vaginal birth or the area from the waist down during a cesarean delivery. They are usually injected along the course of a nerve or nerve bundle and effectively "block" the passage of nerve signals to that part of the body. Regional blocks are better than general anesthesia for a cesarean delivery, because the mother is awake during the birth and alert afterward. During a vaginal delivery, however, they inhibit the mother's urge to push.

The most frequently used regional nerve blocks are epidural, pudendal, caudal, and spinal. *Epidural blocks* (also called *lumbar epidurals*) have become increasingly popular for both vaginal and cesarean deliveries and for relieving severe labor pain. They are relatively safe, because less of the drug is needed to achieve the desired effect and they are easier to administer than the other types of regional blocks. Epidural agents—such as bupivacaine, lidocaine, or chloroprocain—are administered through a tube that has been inserted through a needle into the epidural space (outside the spinal cord). The needle is normally inserted while the mother is lying on her left side or sitting up and leaning over a table to steady herself.

Epidurals are normally discontinued in time to allow the mother to have full control over pushing and are restarted after delivery, when the placenta is being removed or a surgeon is stitching an episiotomy or a cesarean wound. Blood pressure must be monitored continuously when an epidural is used, because these agents can decrease the mother's blood pressure. The mother is given intravenous fluids and medication to counteract this reaction. Leaning the uterus to the left may also help maintain the normal blood pressure. Epidurals usually are not used if the mother starts bleeding or develops placenta previa (when the placenta covers the cervix), severe PIH, or eclampsia, or if the baby shows signs of fetal distress. Sometimes epidurals decrease the fetal heartbeat, which must also be continuously monitored.

Epidurals will weaken your urge to push, which sometimes delays the second stage of labor and can lead to the need for early surgical interventions, such as a forceps delivery, vacuum extraction, or cesarean delivery. So it's important for you to decide in advance under what conditions you will use an epidural. Should any complications develop, your caregiver should discuss all medications with you *before* they are administered.

*Pudendal blocks* are usually reserved for vaginal births (especially for forceps deliveries). The medication is administered through a needle inserted into the perineum while the mother lies on her back with her feet in stirrups. Pudendal blocks are frequently used with pain relievers, such as meperidine. When they're necessary, they are safe and effective.

*Spinal blocks* (for cesarean deliveries) and low spinal (*saddle*) blocks for forceps-assisted vaginal deliveries are administered in a single dose just prior to delivery. The mother lies on her side with her back arched and neck and knees flexed while an anesthetic is injected into the fluid surrounding the spinal cord. There may be some nausea and vomiting while the drug is in effect (about one to one-and-one-half hours). As with epidurals, spinal blocks can decrease the mother's blood pressure. Elevation of the legs, leaning the uterus to the left, intravenous fluids, and medication may be used to prevent or counteract the drop in blood pressure. After delivery, the mother usually remains on her back for about eight hours; a few mothers experience headaches. As with epidurals, spinals are not usually used when there is evidence of placenta previa, PIH, eclampsia, or fetal distress.

*Caudal blocks* are similar to epidurals, except that they block sensation in a more limited area, require a larger dose to be effective, and require greater skill on the part of the anesthesiologist administering them. They can also inhibit labor. Because of these risks, they are used much less frequently than epidurals.

*General Anesthesia*

General anesthesia means the mother is asleep. It is used almost exclusively for emergency surgical births. Because of its rapid effect, it's more likely to be used for an emergency cesarean delivery when there is no time to administer a regional anesthetic. It's occasionally used for vaginal breech deliveries (when the baby's buttocks are in the mother's pelvis).

Inhalants, such as nitrous oxide, are used for emergency deliveries along with other agents to temporarily put the mother to sleep. When she regains consciousness, she may feel groggy, disoriented, and restless. She may also have a cough and sore throat because the anesthetic is given through an endotracheal (in the throat) tube. She may also experience nausea and vomiting and suffer bowel and bladder discomforts. The anesthetic also may cause her blood pressure to fall.

The risk associated with general anesthesia is that both you and your baby are sedated. Sedation of the baby can be minimized by administering the anesthetic as close to the actual birth as possible so that it has little time to cross the placenta barrier in dangerous amounts. Administering oxygen to the mother and tilting her to the side (usually the left side) may also help oxygen reach the fetus.

Another risk of general anesthesia is that the mother may vomit and aspirate (inhale) the vomited material into the lungs, damaging lung tissue and causing complications such as aspiration pneumonia. This is one of the reasons mothers are asked not to eat or drink a lot of liquids when in active labor and why an endotracheal tube is used to administer general anesthetic agents. You may also be given antacids just prior to the procedure to neutralize stomach acid in case you do aspirate.

---

## HOLISTIC GUIDELINES FOR USING PAIN RELIEVERS DURING LABOR AND CHILDBIRTH

Every time you use drugs for pain relief during pregnancy, a very small and vulnerable being inside you may also be affected. Here are some guidelines for using pain relievers wisely during pregnancy and childbirth:

▷ Discuss with your caregiver the smallest dose that will be most effective for the shortest possible time.

▷ Take the medication when it benefits you most—cold medications at night, for instance, to help you sleep.

▷ Follow the package insert or doctor's directions carefully. Some medications must be taken on an empty stomach; some should be taken with food or milk.

▷ Try enhancing the strength of your immune system before resorting to drugs. Take vitamin, mineral, or botanical supplements, eat nutritious foods, get enough rest, and exercise regularly.

# *H*OLISTIC APPROACHES TO COMMON SEVENTH-MONTH CONCERNS

Lower
Abdominal Pain

This month your baby will grow by leaps and bounds! You'll probably feel minor pains in the abdomen as your muscles and ligaments stretch. The pains may feel like sharp, stabbing cramps. They are usually most noticeable when you get up from bed or when you cough. The pain can be brief or last several hours. As long as they are not accompanied by fever, chills, bleeding, increased vaginal discharge, fainting, or other unusual symptoms, there's no cause for concern. Usually you can make the cramps subside by staying off your feet, resting in a comfortable position, or taking a hot bath.

Sometimes your enlarging abdomen causes your abdominal muscles to stretch the skin and cause itchiness and dryness. Be careful not to scratch this area; instead, try a natural lubricating lotion, such as calamine lotion.

*Acupressure*

You can use acupressure to relieve cramps. Try pressing Stomach Point Number 36, which is located three finger widths below your kneecap, in the hollow just in front of the upper aspect of the fibula (the slender bone on the outside of the lower leg). Pressing this point on both legs for several minutes before your main meals may ease digestive cramps.

*Abdominal
Massage*

Gentle massage can relieve abdominal cramps, especially when it's combined with stretching exercises and hydrotherapy. Ask your caregiver to show you how to finger-roll your abdominal muscles, if he or she feels it will help. A simple massage involves using one hand to very gently lift and roll the abdominal muscles in one direction while using the other hand to pull them in the opposite direction. Reversing the direction of each hand establishes a continuous circulation of blood and lymph, which will eliminate temporary cramps.

*Lower Back
Massage*

You can also relieve abdominal cramps by massaging your lower back muscles. The best technique is to gently stroke each side of your spine with the heels of your hands (your fingers should be pointing down and slightly outward). Use the same stroke to massage across the lower back muscles to the hips and buttocks.

## Overheating and Sweating

At times you'll be fanning yourself while everyone else is freezing, or lying flat in bed may make you short of breath and you may notice your heart fluttering (palpitations). This is because your basal metabolic rate increases by 20 percent during pregnancy, causing you to feel overheated and making your heart beat faster. You'll perspire more, particularly at night. Perspiration is good, because it helps cool you off and rids your body of waste products.

If sweating makes you feel uncomfortable, however, try bathing more often, using a natural antiperspirant, and dressing in layers (especially in winter) so that sweat is drawn away from your body and you can peel down to your shirtsleeves when you start heating up. Remember to drink more fluids to replace those lost through sweating. It's extremely important to prevent dehydration throughout your pregnancy.

Chapter *9*

# The Eighth Month

**Y**OU ARE NOW ENTERING YOUR EIGHTH MONTH, and your baby should weigh slightly less than four pounds and be almost eighteen inches long. Most of the baby's systems are now fully developed. Your baby can now see and hear and even recognize your voice.

You may notice that your baby now has identifiable periods of activity and rest. You should feel kicking, sometimes strong enough to wake you up at night. When you lie down, you can probably feel the baby's jerking movements, especially hiccups.

The baby's movements, along with your enlarged abdomen, may cause you to feel a bit clumsy. Most women experience clumsiness and forgetfulness during this month. But don't panic—this is normal. Midwives call this forgetfulness "pregnancy mushbrain." To make sure you remember to take care of all the details of your life, keep lists and write reminder notes to yourself!

## THE EIGHTH-MONTH CHECKUP

After the twenty-eighth week, your caregiver will ask you to come in for a checkup every two weeks. He or she will continue to monitor your weight, blood pressure, your blood and urine, the height of the fundus, the size and position of your uterus, and check for signs of edema and listen to your baby's heartbeat.

You'll want to discuss any new symptoms, including strong, regular fetal activity; increasingly heavy whitish vaginal discharge (leukorrhea); heartburn and indigestion; shortness of breath; stronger Braxton Hicks contractions; and colostrum (a premilk liquid) leaking from your breasts.

## COMMON EIGHTH-MONTH CONCERNS

### Low Birth Weight

Many mothers worry about the birth weight of their babies. Fortunately, these fears are usually not warranted because only 7 out of every 100 newborns are categorized as low–birth-weight babies (weighing less than five pounds, eight ounces), and slightly more than 1 in 100 babies as very low–birth-weight babies (weighing less than three pounds, five ounces).

If you've followed the holistic program outlined in this book, you've avoided the most common causes of low birth weight: tobacco, alcohol, or drug use; poor nutrition; or chronic maternal illness. Even if the baby turns out to be small, the excellent medical care available today will give your baby a good chance of surviving and growing up healthy.

If you think you have reason to worry about having a low–birth-weight baby, talk to your caregiver. A sonogram may be used to determine if your baby is growing at a normal pace. If not, then steps can be taken to discover the cause of the slow growth and, if possible, correct it.

### Premature Babies

Babies are considered premature if they're born before the 37th week of pregnancy. Fortunately, only 9 percent of babies in the United States are born premature. In the past, a baby born before the 28th week had little chance of survival. Today, however, the chance of survival is excellent; even babies weighing less than two pounds can grow up to be healthy adults. Some women believe that sex or a bad fall may cause a premature birth, which is usually not the case. The more likely causes are reduced blood flow to the placenta, an infection in the placenta, uterine tumors, premature membrane rupture, weakness in the cervix, and deformities in the baby or in the mother's uterus. Mothers who conceived using fertility drugs or via in vitro fertilization, who have an increased risk of multiple births, are also at risk of having premature babies because multiple births are usually premature. Twins, for instance, are considered full term (that is, fully developed) at 38 weeks, instead of 40.

If you've followed the holistic prevention program outlined in this book, you've probably done all you can to prevent a premature birth. The most important guidelines are eliminating smoking, alcohol, and recreational drugs, and following the prenatal food plan discussed in Chapter 3.

|  |  |
|---|---|
| ***Botanical Remedies*** | Some midwives believe that raspberry leaf, squaw vine, horsetail, red clover, nettle, echinacea, and goldenseal supplements help prevent premature births. Although there have been no studies on their effectiveness, these supplements are believed to strengthen the immune system. |

Fish oil may also be useful in preventing premature births. The April 1992 issue of the British medical journal *Lancet* reported a study of 533 pregnant Danish women that found that those who took fish oil capsules were more likely to carry their pregnancies to term than those who took olive oil capsules, and their babies appeared to have better vision than otherwise healthy babies born premature.

## Cesarean Births

Approximately 16 to 20 percent of all births in the United States are by cesarean delivery, the surgical operation for delivering a baby by cutting through the mother's abdominal and uterine walls. A cesarean delivery is major surgery and involves a series of separate incisions in the mother's skin, abdominal muscles, and uterus so that the infant can be removed.

There are two types of cesarean procedures—planned and emergency. Planned prelabor cesareans are normally performed at the thirty-eighth or thirty-ninth week to deliver a baby in a footling (feet first) breech position or because the mother has an unusually small pelvis or placenta previa. Planned cesareans may also be recommended during labor if the mother is overly exhausted, her cervix is not dilating, or the baby's heart rate is not normal and her caregiver wants to deliver the baby immediately to prevent further complications.

Emergency cesareans are usually performed only after a mother has started labor and immediate surgery is necessary to deliver the baby because the life of the baby or mother is in danger. A cesarean delivery may last one or more hours, depending on the availability of an anesthesiologist, emergency room, and at least two surgeons. Emergency cesarean deliveries are rare. They are used when there has been a major abruption of the placenta (which could cause the baby to die and the mother to hemorrhage), cord prolapse (when the membranes rupture and the cord falls out), eclamptic convulsions in the mother, or a suddenly dangerous and irreversible fall in fetal heart rate.

There are several different types of cesarean incisions. The most common is a horizontal skin incision just above the pubic bone—the *bikini cut*. This incision is made low in the uterus, where the uterine wall is thinner, so the risk of bleeding is lower, and the risk of rupture in subsequent pregnancies is very low.

Less frequently, a *classical incision* is performed. This is a vertical cut from the navel to the pubic bone. This is usually done only in serious emergencies. A vertical incision allows a larger opening and is used if the fetus is quite large or in a difficult position. The advantage of the classical incision is that it gives the surgeon more room to operate and remove the baby faster.

Classical incisions involve more bleeding and place the mother at greater risk of an abdominal infection. They're usually used as a last resort, because once a mother has had one, it's very unlikely that she'll be able to have a subsequent vaginal birth because her uterus is more likely to rupture along the incision.

Cesarean deliveries are more expensive and require a longer stay in the hospital than vaginal births. In order to make an informed decision, any woman considering a cesarean section should ask her physician to fully explain the benefits, risks, and costs of the operation and its alternatives.

You need to be sure that your caregiver will *not* routinely use the cesarean method to deliver a "breech baby"—where the fetus does not lie in the normal head-first position. Many breech position babies don't require a cesarean, although some obstetricians will perform one automatically unless you discuss the risks and benefits with them prior to going into labor. Many midwives feel that vaginal delivery of certain breech-positioned babies is preferable because cesareans increase the risk of complications for the mother and do not decrease the risk of infant death. If you have a breech baby, ask your caregiver to consider various options before opting for a cesarean, including x-ray–guided pelvimetry, having you rest or walk around, sedating you, or stimulating labor with oxytocin. Even if the baby does not turn, these therapies can speed up labor and encourage the baby to descend, so that it might be able to be born without cesarean delivery. In some cases, there are risks for delivering breech babies vaginally, so be sure your caregiver explains them all to you before you make your decision.

*Medical Risks of Cesarean Births*

Although maternal death during childbirth is extremely uncommon, national figures show that a cesarean delivery carries up to four times the risk of death than a vaginal delivery. Because major surgery is involved, the chance of infection and complication is also greater. The most common are *endometriosis* (when tissue lining the uterus ends up in abnormal locations) and urinary tract or incision infections.

More complications develop during emergency cesareans, usually because they're performed faster and the mother and baby are already having some kind of difficulty. Infants delivered by cesarean, for example, are at greater risk of developing respiratory distress syndrome (RDS) and other lung disorders, or feeding problems.

The best thing you can do to avoid an unnecessary cesarean delivery is to become an informed consumer early in pregnancy. Ask your caregiver how he or she feels about fetal monitoring and what criteria are used to determine when your labor is failing to progress. If you had a cesarean previously, you may also want to know your caregiver's views on trying a vaginal delivery this time. If you want to avoid a repeat cesarean, try to find a sympathetic and supportive caregiver who can help you.

## Vaginal Births after Cesareans (VBACs)

At one time, it was very difficult for women who had a cesarean to later have a vaginal birth. Today, between 50 and 80 percent of women who have had cesareans are able to have subsequent vaginal deliveries. Even women who have had more than one cesarean or are carrying twins have a good chance of being able to successfully deliver vaginally. ACOG guidelines now officially state that repeat cesareans should not be considered routine, and that most women with prior cesareans can have VBACs.

Whether you can have a VBAC depends on the type of uterine incision you had in your previous surgery and the reason your baby was delivered surgically. If you had a low transverse incision (across the lower part of the uterus), as 95 percent of women do today, your chances of having a VBAC now are good. If you had a classical vertical incision (down the middle of your uterus), you will not be able to have a vaginal delivery because of the risk of uterine rupture. If the reason for the cesarean was one that isn't likely to occur again (such as fetal distress, premature separation of the placenta, faulty placement of the placenta, infection, breech position, or toxemia), it's very possible that you can have a VBAC. If the cause was a chronic disease (such as diabetes, high blood pressure, or heart disease) or a structural problem (a badly contracted pelvis, for example), you will probably require a cesarean.

If you feel strongly about having a VBAC, discuss the possibility with your caregiver and ask him or her to review the records of your previous cesarean. For example, some caregivers will not permit a woman with a cesarean-scarred uterus to go through labor. In that case, you will need to find an understanding caregiver who will attend you throughout labor and delivery, and let you labor (called a *trial labor*) as long as possible without medication.

## $\mathcal{U}$NCOMMON COMPLICATIONS

**Incompetent Cervix**

An incompetent cervix is one that dilates prematurely and causes a premature birth. It occurs in 1 or 2 of every 100 pregnancies, and it's believed to be responsible for 20 to 25 percent of all second-trimester miscarriages. Daughters of mothers who were given diethylstilbestrol (DES; a drug used during the 1950s to prevent threatened miscarriages) frequently have incompetent cervices; the causes of incompetent cervices in other women are unknown. No holistic therapies are reported to be able to prevent or treat this condition. It may be the result of genetic weakness of the cervix (the neck of the uterus), extreme stretching or severe lacerations of the cervix during previous deliveries, cervical surgery or laser therapy, or a traumatic D&C or abortion, especially if it was performed when abortions were still illegal.

If an incompetent cervix is diagnosed in time or in a subsequent pregnancy, a *purse-string* suture can be interwoven through the cervix, supporting it and preventing it from dilating too early. Labor can still start prematurely, however, and the suture is usually removed as soon as labor onsets.

## Chorioamnionitis

Chorioamnionitis is an infection of two of the membranes that form the *bag of waters* and contain the amniotic fluid. This may result spontaneously from an infection in the mother crossing the placenta (Group B *Streptococcus* is a common agent.) or through contamination by viral or bacterial agents after the membranes have ruptured. Thus, premature rupture of the membranes is also linked to chorioamnionitis. Chorioamnionitis can cause intrauterine growth (IGR) and stillbirth if it is not detected in time.

Chorioamnionitis is usually detected externally after the membranes have ruptured and an excessive amount of amniotic fluid is present. More often, a baby is not growing normally or becomes ill at delivery, and infection is the suspected cause. Not all infective agents can be identified quickly, however, so your caregiver may think that an infection is involved but may be unable to identify the agent. Treatment depends on the cause of the infection and how the baby is faring.

## Intrauterine Growth Retardation (IUGR)

IUGR is a serious complication in which the baby's growth rate, as measured by fundal height and estimated size (by palpation), slows down. Research indicates that these babies may not be able to withstand labor and that many are irreparably harmed before delivery. Babies born with this condition usually have relatively lower IQs and poor motor skills. Virtually all are born with low birth weights for their gestational age, and most require hospitalization in a neonatal intensive care unit (NICU). Once delivered, however, these babies can gain back their normal weight and develop normally. There are several possible causes of IUGR, including infections, smoking, malnutrition, genetic defects, drug use, or poor blood supply to the placenta due to PIH or detachment from the wall of the uterus.

Fortunately, IUGR can usually be detected during regular monthly checkups. Ultrasound can confirm the diagnosis, in which case the baby's growth can be carefully monitored up until delivery.

## Placenta Previa

Placenta previa is the implantation of the fertilized ovum (egg) near the cervix instead of in the fundus of the uterus. The closer the implantation is to the cervix, the greater the risk of hemorrhaging. Thus, the severity of the condition depends on how much of the cervix is covered by the placenta. This is an uncommon complication that can become an emergency.

Early ultrasound frequently detects marginal or partial previas, in which case the women are often told they must have a cesarean delivery. Prior to the routine use of sonography, placenta previa was normally detected at about the twenty-eighth week of pregnancy, when the mother began bleeding bright red blood. This bleeding is painless at first but becomes progressively more painful and frequent.

In case of a marginal placenta previa, in which a tiny part of the cervix is covered by the implantation, the mother may deliver vaginally without complications. Partial and complete previas usually require a cesarean delivery before onset of labor to reduce the risk of the mother hemorrhaging or the baby dying.

## Placenta Accreta

Placenta accreta is a rare complication in which the placental villi (fingerlike projections of tissue) insert into deeper muscle layers of the uterus instead of just the endometrial (innermost) lining. It is suspected when the placenta does not detach properly after the baby is delivered. It can rapidly progress into an emergency because the mother usually hemorrhages until the placenta is removed. Manual removal under general anesthesia, followed by a D&C, is the normal treatment.

The amount of accreta varies: some attachments can be quite small; others can be extensive. In rare cases, a hysterectomy may be required to prevent further hemorrhage.

## Abruptio Placenta

Abruptio placenta is an uncommon emergency in which a portion of the placenta separates from the uterine wall prior to the baby's delivery. It can occur before or during labor. Severe abruptions are usually accompanied by pain and bleeding and little or no fetal activity. They are normally detected by ultrasound.

Small abruptions may remain undetected, however, even during labor. The greater the degree of separation, the higher the fetal mortality rate. Smoking and malnutrition are the two most common causes of abruption. Some authorities believe that pelvic inflammatory disease (PID) and multiple D&Cs contribute to scarring of the endometrial lining, which can make a woman more likely to experience abruptions.

## Cord Prolapse

Cord prolapse is a rare emergency in which the umbilical cord slips through the cervix ahead of the baby. This usually occurs when the membranes rupture. The baby descends and puts pressure on the cord, pinching it so that the baby does not receive enough oxygen.

Prolapse is more common in babies in breech, footling breech, or transverse positions. The incidence of prolapse is increased by prematurity, polyhydramnios (too much amniotic fluid), and multiple births. Cesareans are required when cord prolapse occurs. The risk of fetal mortality is high, unless a woman can be operated on immediately in a hospital.

## Stillbirths

Children born dead after twenty-two weeks of pregnancy are called *stillborn*. There are several causes of stillbirth, all of which usually involve a loss of oxygen supply to the baby. The most common cause is the formation of blood clots in the umbilical cord, which cut off the critical supply of oxygen-rich blood. A second cause is the premature separation of the placenta from the uterus, which also cuts off the flow of oxygen. Both of these events usually occur during the last three weeks of pregnancy. Finally, the baby's air supply may be cut off if the umbilical cord becomes wrapped around the baby or presses against the pelvis during delivery.

The most common sign of an impending stillbirth is when the mother no longer feels the infant moving inside her womb. Paying close attention to your baby's movements is the best way to detect a sick or dying baby, because active, regular movements are the clearest sign of its well-being. Most mothers of stillborn babies, when questioned later, do not remember when they last felt the baby move. Others tell researchers that they noticed no movement two or three days prior to the stillbirth.

If you notice a sudden change in your baby's activity, especially a lack of fetal movement, report this to your caregiver immediately.

According to many midwives, most mothers of stillborns are aware that their baby has not moved, but due to grief, fear, or denial, they wait too long before reporting it to their caregiver. If reported early enough, many complications can be detected with fetal monitoring, and the baby can be delivered by cesarean section.

## HOLISTIC APPROACHES TO COMMON EIGHTH-MONTH CONCERNS

### Sciatica

In the last months of pregnancy, your enlarging uterus can press against the sciatic nerve—the longest nerve in the body, extending from the low back and down the leg—which may cause pain in the low back, buttocks, and legs. Rest and an ice pack usually help. The pain may pass as your baby's position changes, or it may linger until you've delivered. In severe cases, a few days of bed rest or special exercises (described below) can also be helpful.

### *Breathing Exercise*

This breathing exercise will help relieve nervous tension, ease pain, and relax the muscles around the sciatic nerve. It only takes a couple of minutes and will help you feel relaxed and energized.

**Seated Breathing Exercise**

1. While seated, cross your arms over your stomach. Keeping your middle back pressed against the back of the chair for support, let your chin drop and shoulders roll forward.

2. Start rocking gently, forward and back. As you relax, feel your neck, upper back, and shoulders stretch and expand. To avoid muscle strain, keep your back supported and don't roll too far forward.

3. Breathe deeply as you rock. Allow the rocking motion to find its own pace. It will become shorter and gentler—four to five rocks per breath.

4. Continue rocking for another ten breaths. Slowly straighten up and take a deep breath.

**Standing Breathing Exercise**

1. Place the palms of your hands on the sides of your lower rib cage.

2. Breathe in slowly and deeply to a count of three, so that your hands are pushed apart sideways.

3. Breathe out slowly to a count of four or five, lightly pressing your palms against your rib cage to encourage complete exhalation.

4. Repeat this exercise ten to fifteen times.

*Chiropractic*    A misaligned lower pelvis can sometimes pinch the sciatic nerve. One or two visits to a chiropractor will usually help eliminate the pain.

---

## JOIN THE PEP TEAM!

We discussed fatigue before, but it's worth re-emphasizing the fact that late pregnancy and childbirth are physically and emotionally *draining,* and you need to do everything you can to stay energized. Here are a few more suggestions for keeping your energy level up:

**Posture.**    Poor posture often causes fatigue. If you sit or walk slumped over, your rib cage cannot move as freely as usual and your lungs cannot expand and contract fully. Practice walking with your spine properly aligned.

**Botanical Medicine.**    Take echinacea and goldenseal supplements plus a multivitamin capsule daily, and ask your caregiver about your need for additional vitamin $B_1$, $B_2$, and $B_{12}$ supplements.

**Exercise.**

1. Wake up in the morning by taking a cool shower. Try fresh rosemary crushed into a natural bristle brush for an invigorating scrub massage. This will stimulate your blood circulation for the day.

2. Walk briskly or hike one mile (or as far as you can comfortably) each day.

3. Use the stairs instead of the elevator as often as possible.

4. Do deep-breathing exercises with a few gentle torso twists, then stretch for five minutes.

5. Skip rope lightly for several minutes a day without working up a sweat. This will slowly raise your heart rate and give you more stamina. The effects will last for several hours.

6. Twice a day, stand erect with your back flat against the wall. Clench your stomach muscles below your waist and hold for ten seconds.

**Napping.**    Taking ten-minute catnaps periodically throughout the day will also increase your energy levels. Take them whenever you can—mid-morning, after lunch, just before dinner, or before going out. An excellent napping technique is to put both feet up against a wall to reverse the blood flow, wear eye shades, and listen to relaxation tapes.

**Nutrition.**    Following the nutritional guidelines outlined in Chapter 3 will help you get the calories and nutrients you need for energy. Here are a few more suggestions:

1. For breakfast, sprinkle freshly ground cinnamon on cereal or toast—cinnamon helps metabolize glucose, which is your baby's main energy source.

2. Mix a few crumbled walnuts with several drops of evening primrose oil and poppy seeds, and spread on a slice of whole-grain bread. This snack will give you instant energy and help relax you (walnuts are high in serotonin, which has a calming effect).

3. Drink an eight-ounce glass of water with a few drops of lemon juice or peppermint oil added. Lemon and peppermint scents boost energy levels.

4. Drink eight 8-ounce glasses of water daily. Dehydration is one of the most common causes of fatigue. Try drinking iced carbonated water three times a day.

5. Wait two hours after each meal before having dessert, because simple sugars (even in fruit) are burned quickly for energy and, just as quickly, your energy level may fall.

## Rib Pain

Your growing baby pushes your abdomen into your chest and, as a result, your rib cage has to expand. To do so, the lower ribs must spread out more. This puts a strain on them at the point where they connect with the spinal column or the breastbone (sternum). The strain can produce a considerable amount of discomfort—particularly on your right side—which continues on and off until you deliver. At that time, the rib cage returns to its normal size.

Gentle massage and deep breathing will ease most of the pain. Try placing your palms on your upper chest with your hands slightly apart. Breathe in slowly and deeply to a count of three, filling first your abdomen and then your chest, so that your hands rise noticeably with each inhalation. Breathe out slowly to a count of four, lightly pressing your palms down to encourage complete exhalation.

## Pelvic Pain

In late pregnancy, the cartilage between the pubic bones begins to soften, allowing your pubic joint to expand in preparation for birth. For some women, this expansion causes occasional stabbing pains in the pelvic area. It may worsen after you walk or stand for awhile or when you're tired. You can relieve this pain with hot baths and by periodically lying down with your hips elevated a bit. Positive thinking can help too—keep telling yourself that your body is getting ready for birth and that your baby's head is dropping deeper into your pelvis.

You can also use abdominal breathing to ease the pain. Sit in a firm chair with your feet flat on the floor and your hands palms down on your thighs. Keep your shoulders back and press them slightly toward the floor. Imagine there's a string attached to the top of your head, gently pulling you up. Using your abdomen, breathe in through your mouth, then breathe out, making a soft "fuuu" sound. Imagine the air going up and down your spine through the string as you breathe. Repeat this exercise five to ten times. If you become dizzy, stop.

# ESPECIALLY *for* FATHERS

YOUR ROLE AS A SUPPORT PERSON this month (and next month during labor and birth) is extremely important. You've probably learned a lot about teamwork in childbirth classes, but now is the time to put what you've learned into practice. Your partner may become increasingly anxious about the delivery day and perhaps a bit frustrated, too, because the big day never seems to come fast enough. So give her whatever emotional (and physical) support she needs.

A single massage is worth a thousand words. If your partner has back, leg, or pelvic pain, get out the massage oil. If she's a little down, remind her how wonderful she is. If she's worried about the possibility of complications during birth, remind her that you've both done as much as you can to have a healthy baby. Finally, if she's concerned about the pain of labor and birth, assure her that you'll be there with her every step of the way.

## Chapter 10

# The Ninth Month

GIVE YOURSELF A WELL-DESERVED PAT ON THE BACK! Your ninth month has come, and your baby is now about twenty inches in length and weighs approximately five or six pounds. Baby's nervous system will undergo even more changes this month as he or she grows a fatty sheath, called *myelin,* around nerve fibers. This sheath protects the nerves from damage and speeds up the rate at which nerve impulses travel from one part of the body to the next. The sheathing process is not complete until several months after birth.

## NINTH-MONTH WEEKLY CHECKUPS

After the thirty-sixth week, your caregiver will probably schedule weekly checkups. During these examinations, your caregiver will listen to your baby's heartbeat, estimate your baby's growth and size by palpating (touching) your abdomen, check the body and head position, and look for engagement. Your blood pressure, blood, urine and weight will also be evaluated. These examinations will help you and your caregiver know how close to labor you are. You may spot or bleed after the vaginal exam. If so, discuss this and other concerns with your caregiver.

It's really important that you feel relaxed during this final month before you start labor. Almost everyone has some last-minute questions or concerns. Just make sure you resolve anything that's on your mind by talking it all over with your caregiver.

# COMMON NINTH-MONTH CONCERNS

It took you nine months to grow your baby, and hopefully it'll only take a few hours of labor to give birth. You probably have more questions about the process of labor and delivery than any other aspect of pregnancy. When does labor start? How long will it last? And will I be able to tolerate the pain?

In this chapter, we'll try to answer these questions and help you prepare for labor in advance. As we've said several times, the Holistic Pregnancy Program encourages you to do many relaxation and breathing exercises throughout your pregnancy to stimulate your endorphins naturally. These are your body's natural, powerful pain relievers. The more you do the exercises that release them, the better your chances for not needing drugs during childbirth.

## Premature Labor

*Premature* or *preterm labor* is defined as labor occurring before thirty-seven weeks of pregnancy. It's difficult to predict which women are at risk for preterm labor. Smoking, poor nutritional habits, drug or alcohol abuse, and other poor health practices substantially increase the risk of having a premature or sick baby. If you've followed our Holistic Pregnancy Program (and you don't develop other medical complications), your risk for a premature delivery is pretty small.

If, for some reason, you think you are going into premature labor, call your caregiver immediately. He or she may offer medications that can stop the contractions, giving the fetus more time in the uterus. In severe cases, women may need to be hospitalized or may require emergency care.

One medication approved by the FDA for use during preterm labor is *Yutopar*® (ritodrine hydrochloride), which is given to mothers if labor begins between twenty and thirty-six weeks of gestation and the fetus weighs between 500 and 2,499 grams (one to five pounds). The initial dose is given intravenously, orally, or by intramuscular injection. The amount and frequency of subsequent doses depend on the mother's response to the initial therapy.

According to the FDA, this drug should not be used by women who have cardiovascular disease, PIH, an intrauterine infection, vaginal bleeding, or uncontrolled diabetes. In addition, it shouldn't be used by women with a history of multiple miscarriages due to an incompetent cervix or if your fetal membranes have ruptured. Possible side effects include heart palpitations (fluttering), rapid heartbeat, tremors, anxiety, headaches, vomiting, and fever. Yutopar can also cause blood sugar and bowel problems.

## Premature Rupture of Amniotic Membranes (PROM)

PROM refers to the rupture of the amniotic membranes, or *bag of waters,* before real labor has started. It can occur a few days before the baby is due or weeks—sometimes even months—earlier. Caregivers and hospitals may have different approaches to PROM: Some hospitals may want you to start labor within six hours after PROM; others may want you to wait as long as twenty-four hours.

Researchers still do not know why some women's membranes rupture prematurely. *Collagenase*—an enzyme that breaks down *collagen*, a substance that helps strengthen "stretchable" body tissues—is believed to play a role by reducing the strength and elasticity of the membranes surrounding the fetus. Women who gain more than forty pounds during pregnancy are also at greater risk for PROM. Studies show that maintaining a moderate weight gain and eliminating cigarette smoking—two essentials of the Holistic Pregnancy Program—are the two most important things mothers can do to reduce their risk for PROM.

A vaginal fluid leak—either a sporadic or gushing leak—is an early sign that your membranes may have ruptured prematurely. In most cases, the flow is quite heavy when you lie on your back. Contact your caregiver right away when your membranes rupture.

Some ruptured membranes, especially the sporadic leaking type, heal on their own by resealing. These leaks usually occur high in the amniotic sac and usually only one layer has leaked.

## Position of the Baby

Ask your caregiver to discuss the position of your baby *prior* to delivery. The basic presentations are *vertex* (head first); breech (buttocks first); shoulder (sideways to the pelvis); and frank breech (legs folded flat against the face).

## Breech Positions

If your baby is in a breech position, the head is underneath your ribs and the buttocks are in your pelvis. Many babies assume a breech position at some time during pregnancy. The majority turn head down during the last few weeks; some do so just before birth. Some babies remain in the breech position during delivery and still can be born vaginally without complications. Your caregiver may recommend doing certain exercises during the last eight weeks of pregnancy to encourage a breech baby to turn. If that is unsuccessful, they may attempt to turn the baby manually to a head-down position while it is still in the uterus.

If your baby is still in the breech position at thirty-four to thirty-six weeks, talk to your caregiver about the potential benefit of any of the following methods of encouraging the baby to turn.

### Acupuncture

Acupuncture prior to labor is very effective in turning breech babies. Some acupuncturists give women *moxibustion herbs* to stimulate the acupuncture point on their little toe that's connected to their uterus.

### Physical Activity: The Tilt Position

A midwife also can show you tilt-position exercises that have been used to turn breech babies. You can do this simple exercise twice a day for fifteen minutes each time.

1. Lie on your back with your knees bent and your feet flat on the floor.
2. Raise your abdomen, and prop pillows under your hips so that your knees, hips, and shoulders are in a straight, slanted line.
3. Alternatively, put the wide end of your ironing board on a low couch and lay head down on it.

The baby will not turn while you're doing this exercise; it usually turns while you sleep. It takes at least five days of tilts for the exercise to be effective. If you feel the baby has changed position, call your caregiver to make sure. If it's now head down, stop the tilts.

### Homeopathy

Ask your homeopath to give you pulsatilla formula, which sometimes turns breech babies. Herbal pulsatilla capsules have also been reported by midwives to be very effective.

*Massage*          Massaging your belly often helps. To do so, lie on your back, resting on cushions, so that your hips are higher than your head. Then massage your belly with almond oil for ten minutes, several times each day. Before you start, find out from your caregiver which way your baby is likely to turn so that you can massage in the correct direction.

*Music Therapy*    Restful classical music has also been used by midwives in Canada to turn the baby's head to the down position. Normally, headphones are placed low on the mother's abdomen. Frequently babies will turn toward the sound source. The procedure usually takes five days to be successful. Try it for an hour each day.

*Swimming*         Swimming can help turn a baby's position, although researchers don't know why. Anecdotal evidence from midwives indicates that it may occur due to the double buoyancy of the mother and her baby. One precautionary note: swimming may occasionally turn a vertex (normal) baby, which is small and has plenty of room to maneuver, into a breech. You don't have to worry, however, because this baby will have sufficient room to later turn back to the head-down position.

*Visualization*    According to midwives, visualizing your baby with its head down in your womb can turn a breech baby. They also recommend talking to your baby and explaining that it needs to turn its head down. Frequently, babies who are given such advice turn very quickly.

## PREPARING FOR LABOR AND CHILDBIRTH IN ADVANCE

Every mother eagerly anticipates the birth of her baby, but few look forward to labor. It's hard work. You have an advantage, however, because following the Holistic Pregnancy Program should help you feel physically and emotionally prepared.

Just to be on the safe side, it's a good idea to start practicing your holistic labor exercises now. We hope you'll enjoy the exercises so much that you'll feel totally relaxed and confident throughout your labor. One birthing clinic in London gave women in labor osteopathy, acupuncture, massage, aromatherapy, hypnosis, and breathing exercises while they prepared for labor. Not only that, mothers were encouraged to sit in water tubs, drink small amounts of wine, and listen to classical music. Labor is what you make of it, and we want to help you make it as safe, natural, and spiritual as possible.

## Onset of Labor

Okay, now for the basics. A series of events initiates labor. The most important is that your uterus begins to reduce its production of *progesterone* (the female sex hormone that promotes the transfer of food and oxygen to the fetus and the removal of fetal waste products). This reduction in progesterone usually triggers the onset of labor. Your pituitary gland (a small gland at the base of the brain) will secrete *oxytocin,* a hormone that makes your uterus contract during labor. Your uterus begins to secrete prostaglandins which, like oxytocin, trigger uterine contractions, thereby contributing to the onset of real labor.

Your cervix will dilate slightly before you go into labor. *Dilation* is measured during the vaginal examination by feeling the circular rim of the cervix and estimating in centimeters the diameter of the opening. Many women will be one or two centimeters dilated before they are aware of any signs of labor. During labor your cervix will dilate to about ten centimeters, forming a circle with a diameter of approximately four inches through which your baby will be born.

You probably already know that childbirth is divided into three stages. The *first stage* is dilation of the cervix from zero to ten centimeters; this stage is subdivided into an early, active, and transitional phase. The *second stage* is pushing and delivery, culminating in the birth of the baby. The *third stage* is the delivery of the placenta, or afterbirth. The whole process lasts an average of fourteen hours for first-time mothers and eight hours for women who have already had children. Unless labor is cut short by the need for a cesarean delivery, all women who carry to term go through these three stages. For a very few women, complete dilation passes unnoticed; they don't realize they're in labor until they feel the urge to push, which signals the second (delivery) stage. But this is very rare. Most women definitely know they are in labor.

During labor a woman's uterus will contract as few as 25 times or as many as 300 times. Labor may last a few hours or as long as thirty-six hours. Short labors usually start with contractions that

## SYMPTOMS OF LABOR

The symptoms of labor are divided into subtle signs, preliminary signs, and clear signs.

### Subtle Signs

1. Backaches that may cause restlessness. Different from the posture-related backaches commonly experienced during pregnancy, these backaches are usually caused by early, sometimes unnoticeable, contractions.

2. Several soft bowel movements accompanied by nausea. These are normally caused by an increase in circulating prostaglandins, which cause tissue in the uterus—and along the digestive tract—to contract.

3. "Nesting urge" to clean and tidy. This is a real urge for many pregnant women, but try to resist it. Rest and sleep as much as possible so that you'll be well rested for the upcoming delivery.

### Preliminary Signs

1. You may lose your *mucous plug,* a pink or dark blood-stained clump of mucus from the vagina. This is associated with the thinning of your cervix. It may be seen several weeks before any other signs of labor, or you may not notice it at all.

2. Your "bag" breaks. A small break in your amniotic sac causing minor leakage of fluid without any accompanying contractions. Women sometimes experience periodic leaking of amniotic fluid which is not associated with sponta-

neous labor. These minor preliminary ruptures occur in 10 percent of labors. The leaking usually occurs when you change position, laugh, or sneeze, and may continue off and on for several hours.

3. Continuing contractions that do not progress; that is, they don't get stronger or longer and may even occur closer together. These contractions are called *false* or *prodromal labor.* They help soften and thin the cervix without dilating it. When your cervix becomes riper and ready to dilate, you'll soon be in real labor.

### Clear Signs of Labor

1. Progressing contractions, which last one minute or longer, occur closer together, and hurt more. At this time, the cervix is dilating. Progressive contractions are usually felt in the abdomen and/or lower back. Occasionally women get *leg labor,* usually in their thighs.

2. Breaking of the bag of waters with a pop, gush, or leak, followed by progressing contractions. Labor usually speeds up after the bag of waters breaks. In some women, the membranes don't rupture until very late in labor.

You should learn in advance how to time your contractions by writing down the time each starts and ends. Real labor contractions get closer together, last longer, and become stronger, which means they'll hurt more. Any other pattern indicates false labor.

are fairly close together, about every three to four minutes, and last about one minute each. These can be very painful, as you enter *hard labor* quickly, before your body has had enough time to produce endorphins.

Longer labors usually mean that a mother has an extended prodromal (warm-up) phase with contractions six to twenty minutes apart. This is not *real* labor, but it does help soften and ripen your cervix. Try to rest as much as possible during prodromal labor, and keep yourself well nourished and hydrated. Real labor seldom lasts more than fourteen to eighteen hours. A woman who is in true labor for thirty-six hours usually has complications that may require intervention.

The duration and intensity of labor pains vary from woman to woman. Even in the same woman each labor is different. Some start slowly and then speed up unexpectedly; others start rapidly and then slow down. The amount of pain and fatigue also varies. It's best not to have any definite expectations and to prepare yourself for a wide range of possibilities.

While labor pains can be acute, your body will release endorphins to make them somewhat bearable. Also, the oxytocin in your body can sometimes induce a kind of amnesia. Caregivers have observed, for example, that oxytocin seems to stimulate in women blocks of forgetfulness about their own labor. Relaxing and focusing on breathing and visualization are the key to reducing the intensity of labor pain and increasing your chance of having a shorter, more manageable labor.

## HOLISTIC APPROACHES TO LABOR

Which women have the shortest and least painful labors? One indicator is a woman's stress level during her pregnancy. Women who report more psychological stress during the third trimester of pregnancy tend to have more painful labors. Dr. Grantly Dick-Read, author of *Childbirth Without Fear,* suggests that a mother's stress level in the thirty-second week is a good predictor of the severity of labor pain. That's why we strongly urge you to practice our Holistic Labor Program exercises during your ninth month!

**Relaxation Exercises**

You must be completely relaxed during labor to give your body its best chance of delivering the baby naturally. You should be free to move about, walk, go to the bathroom, lie on your side or back—anything that helps you relax and feel comfortable. Any disruptions may compromise your state of relaxation and can disturb the harmonious process of labor.

Complete relaxation offers minimal resistance to the muscles of expulsion in the birth canal. There are three muscle layers of the uterus. The outer layer runs vertically—up the back, over the top, and down the front—to circle the uterus. These long muscle bands are most prominent in the middle and upper part of the uterus. The middle muscle layer is a mass of interwoven muscles in which the blood vessels lie. The inner muscle layer circles the uterus laterally. These muscle bands are most prominent in the lower part of the uterus and cervix. The outer muscles contract (shorten and tighten) to push the baby down, through, and out of the uterus. The middle muscles contract to squeeze blood into or out of the uterine walls. The inner muscles contract to close the uterine outlet. Thus, the three muscle layers must work synchronously to open the womb and push the baby out. If you're nervous during labor, the inner uterine muscle layer may work against the outer muscle layer, making the delivery of your baby much more difficult.

*Breathing Exercises*

Correct breathing is also essential during labor because the large muscles of the uterus require more oxygen for the amount of work they do, just as a car uses more fuel to go faster or to climb a hill. By breathing more deeply, you'll be better able to supply your uterine muscles with the oxygen they need as well as supply your baby with the nutrient-rich blood he or she will need for life in the outside world.

Practice the following breathing exercise each morning to prepare for labor:

1.  Sitting comfortably, place your hands flat on your lower abdomen with your head up and your shoulders back.

2.  Inhale through your nose, filling your chest slowly with air— filling the upper parts of the lungs, clear up under the collarbones, as well as the lower down to your diaphragm.

3. When you have inhaled as much as possible, let the air out slowly and completely through your mouth. Lean forward slightly, and force out the last possible breath.

Always breathe in through your nose and out through your mouth.

*Guided Imagery Relaxation Exercises*

Have you ever experienced goose bumps while listening to a frightening story or become physically aroused by a sexual fantasy? Then you know firsthand the power of imagery.

Imagery, like visualization, takes advantage of your body's inability to distinguish between vivid mental experiences and actual physical experiences. We strongly recommend that you practice guided imagery exercises during the final month of your pregnancy, prior to labor.

One of the easiest ways to do this is through guided imagery tapes. You can purchase these at many health food stores and some commercial tape shops. Most commercial pregnancy tapes use images such as waves or a flower opening to symbolize labor. You can make your own tape once you've identified the images that relax you and write them into a script. Have someone else record the script, or record it yourself in a soothing voice.

If you've made your own guided imagery tape, it's a good idea to end it with a suggestion such as, "my body knows how to labor." You may feel drowsy after listening to the tape—a good sign, because sleep helps your suggestions sink in.

*Meditation Exercises*

Meditation will help keep you relaxed during labor, and it's a very powerful way of bonding with your baby in the last hours before birth. By meditating, you let your baby know that you're relaxed and that nature is taking its course. There are many different types of meditation. We recommend the following three, to keep you composed, breathing regularly, and focused away from pain.

### Image Meditation

1. Focus your mind on an imaginary object, such as a religious object, candle flame, or a picture of a loved one.

2. At first, your mind will wander to other thoughts. When this happens, gently return to the object of your meditation. With rep-

etition, you'll learn to stay focused on the object for ten to twenty minutes at a time.

### Sound Meditation

1. Focus on a favorite sound and imagine hearing it repeatedly. This can be a sacred word, such as "om" or "ram," or any other sound that makes you feel relaxed.

2. Allow the repetition of the sound to blot out all other thoughts that try to intrude.

3. Eventually, the sound will become blurred and become a droning blanket throughout the meditation period.

### Phrase or Idea Meditation

1. Instead of repeating a sound, focus internally on a repetitive phrase or idea, such as "God is love," or a general idea such as love, truth, or peace.

2. The word, phrase, or idea will help clear your mind of the clutter of thoughts that often cause anxiety and stress.

These exercises might seem somewhat simplistic, but they're used in hospitals and pregnancy clinics and are quite effective. During labor, they can help keep you relaxed and thinking positively.

*Perineal Massage*

It's particularly important to practice perineal massage during pregnancy to prepare the perineum for stretching during childbirth. Perineal massage also reduces scarring and tearing and, thus, the need to have an episiotomy (see Chapter 12).

*Spiral Relaxation*

Spiral relaxation is a variation of progressive relaxation.

1. Lie comfortably in bed, with the palms of your hands facing up.

2. With your eyes closed, imagine a point of light or heat that begins a series of three clockwise spirals around the top of the head and moves down to spiral around the face, neck, upper chest, each arm, the abdomen, hips, thighs, knees, calves, and feet.

3. Let each part of the body relax as the spirals encircle it.

A variation of this exercise can be done lying in bed on your back:

1. Imagine your body being filled with healing energy. Visualize this energy entering through an opening at the top of your head and moving through the frontal lobes, down to the brain stem, and continuing down the length of your spine.

2. Imagine your arms, chest, abdomen, hips, buttocks, thighs, knees, calves, and feet filling with this energy.

3. Allow each part of the body to relax as it is filled with this energy.

*Nutritional Therapies*

Ask your caregiver to recommend a nutritional program for the month prior to labor that will decrease your stress level and increase your energy. Midwives usually advise women preparing for labor to consume more raw or steamed fresh vegetables, whole grains—such as brown rice, oatmeal, and whole-wheat pasta—and a small amount of oily fish, such as salmon, which contain essential fatty acids. They also recommend avoiding coffee and other caffeine-containing substances which can be overstimulating.

*Qigong and Tai Chi*

If you were to go into labor in a Chinese hospital, your caregiver would probably have you practice qigong or tai chi. As discussed in Chapter 1, several forms of these exercises are taught in some hospitals. There are excellent videos that teach simple qigong exercises for pregnant mothers. The simplest is the meditative form, in which you sit in a relaxed pose and use your mental concentration to channel chi to specific parts of your body, especially your womb. This exercise lets you tell your baby that everything is fine and allows you to feel like part of the natural ebb and flow of life.

*Radiant Light Visualization*

Another way of inducing the relaxation response is to imagine yourself being filled with radiant white light.

1. Sit or lie in a comfortable position.

2. Close your eyes. Breathe slowly and deeply for a minute or two.

3. As you inhale, visualize your breath as a radiant white light slowly filling your body. As you exhale, allow your body to relax. Continue for several breaths.

4. Now as you inhale, direct the radiant light to your left foot. As you exhale, imagine the light passing out of your body through the sole of your foot, carrying the tension away.

5. Repeat step 3 as many times as needed, directing the light in turn to each part of your body.

**Humor and Laughter**

You're in luck if your caregiver or labor coach works nights as a stand-up comedian, because laughter—believe it or not—is wonderful therapy throughout labor. Watching a favorite comedy video, TV show, or movie will help you relax. A good laugh, like a good workout, produces an overall sense of well-being, aids digestion, stimulates the heart, and increases the production of endorphins. No kidding!

**Hypnosis**

Hypnosis may help relieve pain during the early stages of labor. A University of Toronto study conducted by Dr. Pamela Letts and reported in the Winter 1993 issue of the *Journal of Women's Health* found that eighty-seven women who practiced deep relaxation exercises (self-hypnosis) experienced milder labor pains than a control group of fifty-six women who were not given any instruction in this technique.

In the study, women were taught self-hypnosis in two office visits. During the first visit, they learned to relax by using soothing imagery and were led through a rehearsal of the delivery process. This helped them learn how to cope with labor one minute at a time. In the next visit, they learned pain control techniques, such as feeling their hands get numb. They were able to transfer the numb feeling to their abdomens during labor.

These are useful exercises to practice on your own now. Letts states that women can easily practice hypnosis/relaxation exercises throughout the day, at home or at work.

**Music**

Researchers have studied the effects of different types of music on relaxation. The most relaxing music for labor will probably have the same rhythm as your heart—about sixty beats per minute. We recommend the slow, second movements of classical pieces, such as symphonies, concertos, or sonatas by Mozart or Beethoven. Meditative New Age music is also used now in birthing clinics.

One stress reduction exercise—tonal massage—involves visualizing musical tones massaging the body. Turn on a favorite piece of music and imagine the tones starting at your feet and moving up your legs and into your abdomen. Visualize the tones relaxing your heart and lungs, slowing down and regulating their rhythms. Visualize the sounds relaxing your shoulders, neck, jaw, eyeballs, and forehead.

# ESPECIALLY for FATHERS

HAVE YOU EVER had a sports injury and were fortunate enough to have a friend rush to your side? Just having a caring presence in your hour of need helped you recover. Multiply this by ten, or perhaps a hundred, and you have some idea of how important you will be to your partner during labor. Studies show that labor and delivery are easier and shorter for women whose partners take part in the process.

If you're taking childbirth classes, you're probably already trained as a labor coach. If not, there are other hats you can wear during this important time. Read through this chapter with your partner, and rehearse the different exercises and massages you may use once her labor starts.

This is an extraordinary event in both of your lives. You can make it truly special by massaging, caressing, relaxing, and inspiring her. This is as close as you can get to the magical creation of life, and you don't want to miss it.

## HOLISTIC APPROACHES TO COMMON NINTH-MONTH CONCERNS

Backaches

Back pain is the most common discomfort immediately prior to or during labor. *Back labor,* as it is called, usually occurs when the baby is in a posterior (*occipitoposterior*) position, with the back of the head pressing against the sacrum (the rear boundary of your pelvis). It's possible, however, to also experience back labor when the baby is *not* in this position or to continue to experience it after the baby has turned from a posterior to an anterior position possibly because the area has become a focus of tension. Here are several holistic measures you can use to relieve this type of pain.

*Acupuncture*

Acupuncture is commonly used in Russia to relieve back labor. One Russian clinical trial of forty-six expectant mothers, reported by Dr. Oscar Oberg in the February 1991 issue of the Russian medical journal, *Akusherstyo i Ginekologiaa,* found that electrical acupuncture was more effective than analgesic drugs in relieving early labor pain. Ask your caregiver if it's all right to have an acupuncturist present during labor.

***Ice Packs and Hot Towels***

Ice packs and hot towels may also ease back pain. Wrap ice cubes in a towel and hold the towel on your lower back. To avoid injury, don't leave it on for more than thirty minutes at a time. Repeat this application hourly. If this does not relieve the pain, try applying hot towels which have been either dipped in hot water or heated in the dryer.

***Massage***

Upper and lower back massage by your partner can also relieve temporary back pain. Ask your partner to try alternating hot and cold compresses with intermittent massaging. The knee-to-chest exercises described in Chapter 4 may also help relieve pain.

## Braxton Hicks Contractions

You may also notice more frequent Braxton Hicks contractions during the ninth month. Some women experience them for the last several months of pregnancy. If you're fatigued and overstressed, these may become more painful, and are one of many reasons for late night "false labor" calls to caregivers. Braxton Hicks contractions are normal and healthy, as they exercise your uterus and stimulate your fetus. They're usually a sign of a good, healthy uterus providing lots of hugs for the baby.

If you begin to experience contractions—painful or not—that occur more than four times an hour or less than fifteen minutes apart, report them to your caregiver or midwife. When they occur, try lying down with your feet elevated, and drink two or three glasses of water or juice. This will usually cause the contractions to subside. If your symptoms do not subside within one hour and you can't get in touch with your caregiver, go to the nearest hospital for further evaluation.

There is no danger that Braxton Hicks contractions will produce real labor even if they're painful. If they annoy you, make yourself a relaxing cup of chamomile tea and lie down in a tub of lukewarm to mildly hot water for one hour.

## WHAT TO HAVE ON HAND AT THE BIRTH SITE

Pack your bag at least three weeks before your due date so that there will be no last-minute panicking. Use the following suggestions as a guide to help you pack.

### Accessories

▷ *Holistic Pregnancy and Childbirth*

▷ 2 pillows for support during labor (hospital pillows are usually skimpy and in short supply)

▷ 1 inexpensive watch to time your contractions (leave your expensive watch and other jewelry at home)

▷ Rolling pin or tennis balls in a sock for back labor. (Fill an athletic sock with two or three new tennis balls and knot the end)

▷ Hot water bottle and frozen camper's ice

▷ Battery-operated tape recorder and music tapes

▷ Contact lenses and glasses

▷ Plastic bags (in case you vomit during labor)

▷ Camera, film, and extra batteries

▷ Lots of loose change for snacks at vending machines and phone calls

▷ Wash cloths and body towels

▷ Hot/cold packs

▷ Infant car seat

▷ Health cards, prenatal records, and copies of your holistic birth plan and monthly checkup forms

▷ Phone book with phone numbers of friends and relatives

### Food

▷ Food and drink for your partner

▷ A cooler filled with chipped ice made from filtered water

### Cosmetics

▷ Lip ointment containing aloe vera and vitamin E

▷ Massage oil containing aloe vera and vitamin E

▷ Premoistened makeup remover (which removes makeup and moisturizes the skin at the same time)

▷ Toiletry items (trial-size products of your favorite soaps, bath and shower gel, and shampoos)

▷ Make up (optional)

### Clothes

▷ Loose clothes (remember that you won't be back to your pre-pregnancy size right after giving birth)

▷ Nursing bra or a comfortable sports bra

▷ Slippers (pack a pair that slip on and off easily); for cold climates, use booties made of sheepskin and breathable fleece

▷ Warm socks

▷ Robe

▷ 1 nursing gown that buttons up the front or has built-in breast flaps for easy access for your nursing baby

▷ 1 going-home outfit for yourself

▷ 1 going-home outfit for your baby, including diapers, undershirt, hat, and blanket

### *Holistic Medicine*

▷ Homeopathic remedies approved for labor, delivery, and postpartum

▷ Approved Bach flower remedies

▷ Approved botanical medicine

Well, the nine months are almost up and you're nearly there—only a few more hours before you bring your child into this world. Those few hours can be frustrating and tiring—unless you're prepared. We hope that this chapter has helped you tap into the natural, holistic ways of stimulating your body's own painkillers. We'll give you even more helpful tips in the next chapter. Your big day is fast approaching!

Chapter *11*

# Labor and Birth

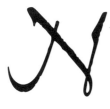ine months of exercise, careful food choices, and all those relaxation exercises have finally paid off. The first stage of labor will soon begin.

As you already know, during the first stage of labor your cervix will begin to efface (thin) and dilate to four or five centimeters. Your contractions during this stage may not feel strong at first, but they will become longer, stronger, and closer together with time.

Most low-risk, first-time mothers whose contractions begin slowly and then gradually accelerate can plan on spending the first several hours of labor at home. But if your contractions start off strong, last at least forty-five seconds, and occur more often than every five minutes, your first several hours of labor may well be your last. Chances are that much of the first stage of labor passed painlessly, and your cervix dilated significantly during that time. You should be timing your contractions and jotting down both their frequency and duration, because your caregiver will need that information later.

## WHEN TO CALL YOUR CAREGIVER

Some women experience very irregular contractions. If you're having strong, long (forty- to sixty-second) contractions, don't wait for them to become regular before calling your caregiver or heading for the hospital. No matter what you've heard or read, it's possible that your contractions are about as regular as they are going to get and that you're well into the active phase of labor. When you call your caregiver or birth site to tell them you're in labor or to ask for advice, be sure to tell them if your water has broken or if you've had a *bloody show* (which indicates that your cervix has begun to dilate actively), how long and how many minutes apart your contractions are, how strong or painful they feel, and what kind of fetal activity you can detect.

If you're within a week or two of your due date, you should probably wait for absolutely clear signs of active labor before going to the hospital (see Chapter 10 for a refresher on these), unless your bag of waters seems to be leaking. If your pregnancy has been complicated with diabetes, high blood pressure, or other medical conditions, or if you're carrying twins or a breech baby, your doctor may advise you to go to the hospital as soon as possible. If you're several weeks away from your due date, call your caregiver. Your contractions may indicate early or premature labor, which can often be stopped if treatment is initiated early enough.

There are different types of labor patterns, each determined by the cycle of your contractions. Prodromal (latent) labor is not uncommon. These contractions are more than five minutes apart (usually ten to fifteen minutes apart) and usually last fifteen to thirty seconds. Normally, very little dilation occurs. You should rest as much as possible during this stage, eat lightly, and keep well hydrated. This phase can last a long time for some women, especially if the cervix has not yet thinned. Try to see prodromal labor as your body's way of preparing for harder labor.

In *early active labor,* you have contractions every five minutes or less with each one lasting at least one minute. If you're a first-time mother, your cervix must thin out (efface) completely before you dilate fully. Mothers who have already given birth usually efface and dilate simultaneously.

Although this is good labor, it will rarely cause dilation beyond three to four centimeters. This is sometimes called the *learn-to-labor* phase. You'll find that the contractions are increasingly painful. The important thing is to immediately start breathing and relaxation exercises, which release your body's endorphins. Breathe for every contraction.

# *H*OLISTIC APPROACHES TO THE FIRST AND SECOND STAGES OF LABOR

It's important to rest and, preferably, sleep during the early stages of labor to conserve your energy. If you can't sleep, don't lie in bed timing contractions—this will only make labor seem longer. Get up, exercise, do relaxation exercises, massage yourself, keep lists, play games, and otherwise divert yourself from thinking about your contractions.

## Latent Phase

**Hot Baths or Showers**

Take a warm bath (but only if your membranes haven't ruptured) or shower and use a heating pad if your back is aching. Don't take aspirin or lie on your back. Lying on your back hurts more, and psychologically, it makes you feel more helpless. In some cases, it can also cause your uterus to press against a major artery and lower your blood pressure (hypotension). It's better to sit up or walk around to increase the effect of gravity on your descending fetus and encourage labor.

**Nutrition and Supplements**

Eat a light snack (broth, toast with apple butter, or fruit juice) if you're hungry. Don't eat a heavy meal, especially if it includes hard-to-digest foods, such as meats, milk or milk products, and fats. Not only will digesting a heavy meal compete with the birthing process for body resources, but a full stomach could cause complications if you need anesthesia later on. It will also make it more likely that you'll vomit.

## Active Labor

Once contractions are three minutes apart or less and last at least one minute, you're in active or *hard labor*. These are real labor contractions, not false labor. Once you've reached four centimeters, dilation normally speeds up. During this phase, your baby descends further into the pelvis and induces full dilation.

Walking, kneeling, standing, or sitting in different positions can help ease the pain of contractions. You should now be doing your breathing and relaxation exercises constantly, experimenting to find what works best for you.

The active phase of labor usually lasts an average of two to three and a half hours. As your contractions become stronger, longer (forty to sixty seconds long, with a distinct peak at about half that time), and more frequent (three to four minutes apart, although the pattern may not be regular), your cervix will dilate to about seven centimeters. You'll have less time now to rest between contractions. You will feel more uncomfortable during contractions, and will probably be unable to talk through them. You may also experience lower back pain, leg discomfort, fatigue, and increasing vaginal blood. You may experience all of these symptoms or just one or two. Your water may break now if it hasn't already.

Drinking clear beverages or Gatorade® to replace lost fluids will help keep your mouth moist. If you're hungry, you should snack on nonfat, low-fiber foods, such as sorbet, a gelatin dessert, or applesauce. If your caregiver or hospital prohibits anything else, sucking on ice chips will help you cool off (your body temperature will increase during labor and consequently you'll sweat more), although some women find that ice chips make them nauseous.

## Advanced Active or Transitional Labor

Transition is the most exhausting phase of labor. The contractions are now more painful, occurring every two to three minutes and lasting sixty to ninety seconds, with very intense peaks that last for most of the contraction. You may feel as though the contractions never completely disappear and that you can't completely relax between them. The final three centimeters of dilation, to the full ten centimeters, will probably take place in a very short time, usually within fifteen to sixty minutes.

In transition, you'll feel a lot of pressure against your lower back, perineum, and rectum, which may cause you to grunt involuntarily. You may feel very warm and sweaty or chilled and shaky—or alternate between the two. You'll bleed more as more capillaries in the cervix rupture. Your legs may feel sore and cold. You may become nauseous and drowsy—which is not surprising, considering how hard you're working! Try to focus your energy with self-hypnosis, imagery, visualization, or meditation exercises learned in this book to keep yourself thinking and feeling positive.

## SECOND STAGE OF CHILDBIRTH: PUSHING AND DELIVERY

The second stage of childbirth, pushing and delivery, begins when you're fully dilated at ten centimeters and feel an irresistible urge to push your baby out the birth canal. Your contractions will last about sixty to ninety seconds and occur two to five minutes apart. There is usually a well-defined rest period between contractions, although some women have trouble recognizing the onset of each contraction.

Depending on your physical fitness, you may experience a burst of renewed energy or increased fatigue. You'll probably be able to see your uterus rising noticeably with each contraction. You should be able to push three times now with each contraction. You'll also bleed more and feel a burning, stinging sensation in your vagina as the baby's head begins to crown.

Once you feel pushing urges, your baby will usually be born in one to two hours. Second-time mothers usually deliver their babies within ten minutes to one hour of feeling the urge to push. You'll know when the head starts to crown—it will feel slippery and wet as it emerges. Try to look down or use a mirror to watch your baby enter the world. It's an incredible, magical moment that you don't want to miss.

## Pushing Techniques

Your caregiver will encourage you to push according to your own urges. This is called *physiological pushing*—long, strong pushes for big urges; short, gruntlike pushes for mild urges. Each uterine contraction, along with your bearing-down efforts, will push the baby closer to the opening of the birth canal. Change your pushing position every thirty minutes—it helps move your baby down the birth canal. Try semi-sitting, side-lying, squatting, or kneeling.

Your uterus does 80 to 85 percent of the actual work of expelling your baby; your pushing adds the other 15 percent, but that 15 percent is crucial. The best way to push is only when you have to. There will be intense rectal pressure and, usually, lower back pain. You'll feel the baby move ahead with a push, then slide back. This "two steps forward, one step back" action is actually good for the baby, since it gently forces fluids from your baby's lungs, gently stimulates its nervous system, and stretches your vagina.

### Recommended Way of Pushing

1. Breathe slowly until the urge to push establishes itself.

2. Take a fast, deep breath, hold it, then drop your jaw, round your shoulders, and push.

3. Push only as long as is necessary during the bearing-down urge.

4. Breathe deeply and relax between contractions. The urge will re-establish itself.

5. Repeat the process.

6. Remember to keep your mouth and jaw open and relaxed so that your vaginal muscles stay relaxed as well.

It may take twenty contractions until you've learned to push well. Eventually, the baby's head will not recede during contractions, and you will feel a stretching, burning sensation as the head crowns. Your caregiver may at some point tell you not to push. You will still feel your uterus pushing, however. Don't try to add a push. Blowing or panting will help you fight the urge to push.

The best time to push is when your body makes it happen—only when the urge to push occurs. That way you won't hold your breath so long that you or your baby get too little oxygen.

As the baby's head is born, and later the shoulders, your caregiver may ask you to pant gently to avoid pushing too hard. This will help prevent any sudden or excessive pressure on the outlet and help prevent tearing.

## Relaxing between Contractions

In general, you should stay upright and active as long as possible. You can walk around, stand, kneel, or sit upright until you feel it's too uncomfortable. You can then lie down—but not on your back. Gravity helps your baby descend, so walking and standing help increase the strength of contractions, ease the pain, and help the baby enter the world. Upright positions move the baby off your back and deeper into your pelvis, thereby reducing pain. Upright positions may also help you feel more in control and reduce any fear and stress, which could make the pain worse.

Whatever position you choose, it's important to relax fully between contractions. Also remember to change positions every twenty to thirty minutes. Have your partner or labor coach remind you when twenty minutes has expired, as you may not be aware of time. Drinking fluids will help your contractions. Sports drinks help replenish your electrolytes stores. Avoid orange and apple juice, because they can cause vomiting. Water and ice chips are fine, although they don't contain the energy calories of Gatorade.®

You should also try to urinate every hour. This will motivate you to change positions when you really don't feel like moving.

Eventually you may find lying down necessary. Fatigue and the sensation of the baby deep in your pelvis at 8 centimeters will help you relax in bed.

**Hot Packs or Ice Packs**

You may find that hot packs on the lower portion of your abdomen help ease the pain of contractions. Some women find cold packs on the lower part of their back helpful. Rubbing a cool, moist washcloth over your face and neck also will feel relaxing. Being touched and rubbed, especially in tense, sore areas, such as the shoulders and lower back, will also be helpful. If you feel a bit out of control, have your partner firmly hold your hand and do your breathing exercises with you.

**Squatting Exercises**

Many childbirth educators encourage women to learn to squat during labor. By squatting, you open your pelvis and give your baby more room to descend. Sitting on a bedpan may help if you find it difficult to relax; toilets and birthing stools also simulate squatting and are more comfortable. Some hospitals and birth centers provide squatting bars. Some mothers report that they found it helpful to sit on a birthing stool placed in warm water during labor. You should discuss all of these alternatives with your caregiver.

Semi-sitting works well for some women, especially during delivery. This position has the added advantage of giving your caregiver good access to your baby and allowing you to see your baby emerging more easily. Lying on your side is also comforting.

## Delivery

Once your baby's head begins to emerge, you'll feel a stretching or burning sensation in your vagina. Your caregiver will probably tell you at this point not to push too hard, because sudden pushes can make the baby come out too quickly and tear your perineum. Try rapid, pantlike breaths so that the baby exits slowly. Once the baby's head is born, it will turn to one side. The shoulders will come out and, finally, the rest of the body.

The baby should be laid on your abdomen for breastfeeding; the cord is normally long enough to reach, so you can begin breastfeeding before it's cut. Before laying the child on your abdomen, your caregiver will quickly suction the baby's nose and mouth to remove excess amniotic fluid and mucus. This is normally done with a rubber bulb syringe or a little jar and tube called a *mucus trap*. Suctioning is done only if the baby's airway seems to be congested or if your baby was under stress during labor and breathing problems are anticipated. The only other cleaning necessary is a gentle washing off of any blood or *meconium*—the baby's first bowel movement. The normal *vernix caseosa,* which is the whitish, cheesy deposit covering your baby's skin at birth, shouldn't be removed, because it protects the baby from skin infections until it is absorbed by the baby's skin. Not all babies have much vernix. For some babies, it's hardly noticeable.

Your baby's umbilical cord will then be clamped in two places close to the abdomen. If your partner is present and wants to, he can cut it. Although cutting the cord releases a spurt of blood, neither you nor the baby will feel it, since there are no nerve endings in the cord. Your baby will then be dried off with soft towels, and wrapped in a warm blanket with its head covered.

## Bonding and Breastfeeding

Years ago, it was common practice for doctors to give women breastfeeding suppressors after birth, assuming they would bottle feed. While this is unlikely to happen today, it is a good idea to be sure you understand the purpose of everything you are asked to take. If you have any doubts about safety for you and your baby, do not hesitate to ask questions. You may even want to ask your partner to be vigilant about asking questions on your behalf, since you will understandably be thinking of other things just after your baby is born.

It's very beneficial if you can hold your baby as soon as he or she is delivered and nurse before the baby is given eye prophylaxis (usually erythromycin ointment). Your baby will start suckling as soon as he or she latches onto your breast. Most infants will imitate crawling motions toward the breast immediately after delivery and suckle in less than an hour, provided they are not drugged or disturbed.

Bonding with your baby by breastfeeding or massage and cuddling is not only an important spiritual event, it also has immediate medical benefits. According to Victoria Schneider, a midwife, babies who are simply touched and massaged immediately after birth gain more weight. In addition, massaging your newborn helps reduce stress levels in you and your baby. A University of Miami Medical School study found that after a thirty-minute massage, both the mothers and their babies had lower levels of cortisol and norepinephrine (stress hormones) and were more alert, less restless, and better able to sleep. So, if possible, massage or nurse your baby as soon as he or she is delivered. You're the most important person in your baby's life. Just feeling your reassuring and gentle pats, nursing, and hearing your familiar voice will provide early nurturing and reassurance.

***Apgar Test***      Once your baby is warm, your caregiver will administer the *Apgar test,* which assesses the baby's development. Each of the five Apgar signs are rated on a scale of zero to two, with ten being the best possible total score. Scores of seven to ten indicate that your baby is in good condition. If the total score is below seven, your baby may need to be taken to the nursery for more observation and care.

Within the first hour after birth, your baby will receive eye medications—either erythromycin or tetracycline (both antibiotics) or silver nitrate. These are usually required by law and given to prevent eye infections, which can cause blindness. Many women prefer the antibiotic ointments over silver nitrate, since they do not burn or irritate the baby's eyes as silver nitrate does.

## A P G A R   S C O R I N G

| Sign | No Points | One Point | Two Points |
| --- | --- | --- | --- |
| Heartbeat | None | Slow (below one hundred beats per minute) | One hundred beats per minute or more |
| Breathing | None | Slow, irregular breathing and weak cry | Good, strong cry |
| Muscle tone | Limp | Some flexion (bending) | Active movement of arms and legs |
| Reflex | No reaction | Grimace | Lusty cry |
| Color | Blue-gray, pale | Normal skin color, except bluish hands and feet all over | Normal skin color when suctioned |

# THIRD STAGE OF CHILDBIRTH: DELIVERING AFTERBIRTH

Once you've nursed and held your baby, your caregiver will guide you through expelling your placenta, which usually takes five to thirty minutes. The normal procedure is for your caregiver to keep one hand on your abdomen to determine when the placenta separates from the wall of your uterus. You will then be asked to push the placenta out. You may feel slight cramps, but usually there is very little discomfort.

Don't be surprised if you continue to have mild contractions. This is due to squeezing of the uterus to separate the placenta from the uterine wall. It also controls hemorrhage from the placental site and moves the placenta into the vagina so that you can push it out.

For most women, delivering the placenta is easy—it usually slides right out. You will be so engrossed with your baby that being asked to push again (usually just one additional push) is not difficult, although you may have some pain if you had an episiotomy or severe tearing.

It's important that your uterus remains contracted to minimize bleeding (it will bleed *more* if it is relaxed). Most women lose about one cup of blood during this time. If your caregiver thinks that you're losing too much blood, he or she may massage your uterus vigorously or ask you to stimulate your nipples to stimulate contractions. In extreme cases, your caregiver may inject you with Methergine® (methylergonovine) or Pitocin (oxytocin), which will cause your uterus to contract. He'll also check your vagina to determine if you need stitches. If you had an episiotomy, the incision will be quickly stitched closed.

You need to stay focused and alert, as there are still small tasks that you'll need to attend to. If you had a hospital birth, you may be moved from the delivery room to the postpartum ward (if you delivered in the Labor Delivery Recovery Postpartum (LDRP) room, you'll probably stay there). Ideally, your partner and family members will be with you, so they can run errands and make your move easier.

One thing you can do for a quick energy boost is your abdominal deep-breathing exercises (you should be doing them anyway to deliver the placenta). A sports beverage will also give you energy.

Have your partner massage you with cool towels dipped in red raspberry, comfrey, or aloe teas; it will stimulate your circulation and refresh you. Virtually anything goes better with a brisk, lovely smelling massage, even childbirth!

*Examination of Your Baby*

Besides the Apgar tests, a more thorough physical examination of your baby will be done several hours following birth. Make sure your caregiver knows that you would like to be with your baby during the exam. The exam normally includes a thorough checkup of all the baby's systems, including the toes; the fontanels (soft spots at the top and back of the head); the eyes, ears, nose, mouth, and throat; the ability to suck and swallow; the size of the head; the weight and length; the breathing pattern; the size of the liver and spleen; the heart tones and lung sounds; the genitals; the hip joints; the overall appearance; and the baby's reflexes. Footprints and handprints may also be taken. The baby's temperature, feeding patterns, activity levels, breathing and heart rate patterns, and urination and bowel movement patterns will also be checked.

Your baby then will be given a vitamin K shot to promote normal blood clotting. Because babies are not born with enough vitamin K for the first few days after birth, this is an important preventive treatment. Your baby's skin will also be examined for any marks. If your baby has a slightly yellow skin color several hours following birth, he or she will be evaluated for *jaundice* (see Chapter 12). Your caregiver may want to measure the blood level of *bilirubin* (a by-product of the breakdown of red blood cells) by drawing a blood sample (usually via a heel prick).

*Circumcision*

If you had a boy, most hospitals will recommend that he be circumcised (have the foreskin of his penis cut back). Studies have shown that urinary tract infections are ten times more common in uncircumcised than circumcised boys. The American Academy of Pediatrics officially recommends that all male babies be circumcised. Your caregiver may advise against it if they think it might cause excess pain, hemorrhaging, infection, or surgical trauma.

# ESPECIALLY *for* FATHERS

HOLISTIC FATHERS ARE WHOLEHEARTEDLY HELPFUL FATHERS—and what you can do to assist your partner (and baby) during childbirth is only limited by your interest, childbirth training, and your chosen birthing site. Your most important function is to make sure your partner feels safe, relaxed, comfortable, and confident. If you've taken childbirth classes and are the labor coach, you're probably already looking forward to helping her throughout labor with her breathing and relaxation exercises; massaging her abdomen, back, neck, and legs; and otherwise keeping her relaxed.

After reading this chapter, you'll probably think of other ways to help out, such as reminding her to urinate at least once an hour, making sure she has an ample supply of ice chips to suck on or fluids to sip, and playing soothing music. Until pushing starts, try distracting her with card games, conversation, encouragement, and support between contractions. Help her change positions, walk around with her, and help her do exercises that may ease her pain, help her pass the time, and speed up labor. Communicate any concerns she may have to her caregiver, especially concerns about your Birth Plan. Once labor starts, encourage her to push, and breathe with her. Help her relax between contractions with soothing words; a cool cloth applied to forehead, neck, and shoulders; and a back massage to help ease back pain. Support her back while she's pushing—hold her hand, wipe her brow, and do whatever helps her.

## Chapter 12

# First Week Postpartum

*Y*OU NOW HAVE A BRAND NEW BABY!

If you had a normal vaginal delivery, you should be back home within forty-eight hours, nursing your baby and surrounded by flowers and baby cards. Don't be surprised if you're too preoccupied with basic body functions (urination, bowel movements, vaginal discharge, breastfeeding) to smell the flowers. At first, it may seem as though every opening in your body has something coming out or going in.

Fortunately, you've had a nine-month boot camp in holistic medicine and you know how to get those endorphins going. You know so much about generating those little neurochemicals that you can do it in your sleep. Which is a good idea, by the way. While you're resting, make a mental affirmation that you will heal as quickly and completely as possible. Visualize white light filling your body with healing energy (see Chapter 4).

You need to recover as quickly as possible, for your own health and happiness and to nurse and bond with your baby. Since holistic medicine is all about self-healing, this chapter discusses holistic approaches to common postpartum concerns, as well as postpartum exercises and tips for successful breastfeeding and basic baby care.

# Mom's Postpartum Checkup

How often you see your caregiver for postpartum checkups will depend on your condition and that of your baby. Usually, mother and baby see the caregiver on the first, third, fifth, and tenth day after delivery, but this will vary. You may want to continue seeing your caregiver and have your baby examined by a pediatrician.

During the first week postpartum, depending on the type of delivery you had, you may experience bleeding *(lochia)*, exhaustion, fever, perineal pain and swelling, difficulty urinating, bowel discomfort, breast engorgement, and depression. Keep a list of your symptoms (use your Postpartum Checkup Form) and any unusual pain, and discuss them at your first checkup.

A lot of mothers assume that they'll be out of commission for several weeks, and lie back and *wait* for healing to set in. We encourage you to take the initiative and begin to help yourself heal right after delivery. Giving birth is a natural process—the body instantly expects to heal itself. You can heal very quickly if you use the combination of holistic therapies we discuss in this chapter.

# Baby's Postpartum Checkup

During the baby's first checkup, your caregiver (or pediatrician) should assess the following:

▷ General appearance: cleanliness, nutrition, alertness

▷ Skin: color, rashes, bruises, swelling, condition of hair and nails

▷ Eyes: eye movement, response to light, vision

▷ Ears: condition of ear canal (evidence of irritation or infection of the ear canal or eardrum)

▷ Nose: condition of passageways (evidence of congestion or discharge)

▷ Mouth: condition of gums, tongue, throat, tonsils

▷ Neck: size of thyroid gland and lymph nodes

▷ Heart: rate and rhythm

▷ Lungs: respiration rate, abnormal noises, air exchange

▷ Abdomen: bowel sounds, tenderness

▷ Arms and legs: movement and color

▷ Hips: normal placement of infant sockets

▷ Pulse: equal femoral pulses

▷ Neuromuscular: muscle tone, movement and coordination, and strength; reflexes

## HOLISTIC APPROACHES TO MOM'S POSTPARTUM SYMPTOMS

**Bleeding (Lochia)**

During the first three days postpartum, you may see bright red fresh blood (as much as a pint for all three days) coming from the vagina. When you stand, you may pass fresh red blood as well as blood clots; this is normal. Beginning the second day postpartum, the bleeding will be more like a heavy period. Every day thereafter, the bleeding should become lighter and less red. Eventually it will turn pink, brown, or yellow. Lochia can last up to six weeks, although most women find that it ends by four weeks postpartum. Nursing helps to shorten the bleeding period; uterine massage works as well.

*Massage*

Massage your uterus to ensure that it stays contracted and begins to shrink, as this helps to control bleeding. The first day after delivery, your uterus should feel firm and about the size of a grapefruit. It should be below the level of your navel. Your caregiver will show you how to check and "rub down" your uterus.

**Afterpains (Uterine Cramps)**

You may experience cramplike abdominal pain, especially if you're nursing. This is caused by contractions of the uterus as it makes its normal shift back into the pelvis following birth. The cramps are more likely if your uterine muscles are flaccid because of previous births or excessive stretching. If cramping is severe, your caregiver may give you analgesics. If they persist for more than a week, you should call your practitioner to rule out other problems, including an infection.

Midwives usually recommend taking one or two tablets of acetaminophen (Tylenol) to relieve discomfort. They also advise visualizing energy flowing through your uterus and down your legs to your toes. Try curling up with a pillow, putting hot towels on your stomach, and letting the baby nuzzle against you.

## Cesarean Pain

Immediately following a cesarean delivery, you shouldn't feel too much pain, because the epidural used during surgery remains effective for several hours. Some hospitals have "patient-administered pain pumps," which release pain relievers through an IV line when you press a button. The catheter and IV lines are uncomfortable, but they will be removed within eighteen to twenty-four hours following birth, after which you'll be given meperidine. Once your bowels sounds can be heard by stethoscope, you will be able to start consuming liquids, then semisolids, and, finally, whole foods.

If you have a private room, your partner may be allowed to stay with you during recovery. You may not feel like nursing your baby because of the pain, in which case most midwives recommend taking mild analgesics to help you nurse. It can also help a lot to place a pillow over your stomach while the baby lies on it nursing.

Second-time cesarean mothers seem to have less trouble adjusting to the pain and emotional stress of surgery. For one thing, they are familiar with their pain threshold. They also normally feel much less pain, because nerves in their abdominal and muscle walls have already been severed during previous births. Beginning on the fourth or fifth day postpartum, however, your uterine nerves will begin to regrow, and you may feel short, stabbing pains (as though they're being "picked" inside) when you sneeze or cough. Nursing can help, because it produces endorphins which will ease these pains. Be careful not to pull or strain your stomach, abdominal, or vaginal muscles while sleeping. Try sleeping on your side supported by large pillows.

## Perineal Pain and Swelling

Your perineum may be sore and swollen for several days after birth due to stretching, bruising, or suturing. If your delivery was suture-free and you've been massaging your perineum regularly, you shouldn't feel excessive pain, and any bleeding should be minimal.

Whether you tear or not will depend on several factors: whether you have pliable, well-nourished tissues; the size of your baby; and your caregiver's ability to help you push correctly during labor. If internal muscles were cut during your episiotomy, or you had severe tearing, you'll need suturing.

You can apply ice packs and take Tylenol to relieve any pain. The pain will lessen every day, although day four or five will be most uncomfortable because severed nerves start to regrow at that time.

Do not douche or use tampons during this period, as they can cause infections.

**Botanical Medicine**

Murray and Pizzorno's *Encyclopedia of Natural Medicine* suggests that *bromelain* (an enzyme found in pineapple) supplements may help reduce swelling and inflammation. They cite a double-blind trial of 160 women who had episiotomies, which found that those who took bromelain supplements had less swelling and pain than those who took a placebo. They suggest that bromelain helps break up proteins into easy-to-assimilate amino acids that they claim will prevent and ease cramping, and also help reduce high blood pressure.

**Baths**

Taking a warm water bath at twenty-minute intervals is also helpful. Witch hazel or essential oil of lavender applied to a sanitary napkin also can help reduce swelling.

**Kegel Exercises**

The Kegel exercises outlined in Chapter 4 will help ease pain, because they stimulate circulation and help reconnect severed nerve pathways.

**Physiotherapy**

If you've had an episiotomy or severe tearing, you may find it difficult to walk without pain. Physiotherapy will help you relearn how to walk in a relaxed and comfortable way. Physiotherapy also restores the circulation of blood in abdominal muscles and reduces swelling and pain. If you plan to give birth in a hospital or birth center, ask your caregiver if they have a physiotherapy program; these usually combine exercise, massage, and relaxation exercises.

## Fatigue

Giving birth is the equivalent of running a marathon, so nobody can blame you if you feel *exhausted*. Try the holistic remedies for fatigue outlined in Chapter 2; namely, acupuncture, acupressure, aromatherapy, Ayurvedic herbs, Bach rescue remedy, biofeedback, botanicals (alfalfa, dandelion, nettle, red raspberry, and comfrey), chiropractic, and homeopathic medicines. Sports drinks may also help give you energy. So will getting as much rest as you can.

## Fever

Your body temperature may be slightly elevated (up to 100°F) for a few days after birth, usually due to hormonal changes and *let down* (your milk coming in). If you have a temperature higher than 100°F, there's a slight chance that you have an infection, which your caregiver should monitor closely. Although infections are uncommon, your caregiver can give you antibiotics which are safe for you and your nursing baby. If you don't have an infection, your immune system may need gentle strengthening, so ask your caregiver about taking echinacea, goldenseal, or feverfew supplements.

## Painful Urination

You may find it difficult or painful to urinate the first week postpartum. Starting Kegel exercises after the first day will help. Make sure you keep your perineum clean after urination; an excellent method is to spray it with warm water using a spray bottle. Also, try urinating

# Especially for Fathers

THE POSTPARTUM PERIOD IS A TIME OF ADJUSTMENT. It will take time for your partner to regain her normal strength. She may have light bleeding (like a period) for four to six weeks, and she may be very sore from stretching or suturing. Her breasts will also be sore and tender, whether she's breastfeeding or not. If the baby was born by cesarean section, the incision on her abdomen will also be very sensitive. She may experience mood swings and postpartum depression, as well. These usually disappear after six to eight weeks. If they don't go away, encourage her to contact her caregiver.

Most of your partner's time during the first few weeks will be spent caring for the baby. You can begin bonding with the baby, as well, by helping to change diapers and burping, and spending lots of time cuddling the baby. Remember: nothing helps bonding more than a good massage! And don't forget to share in the feeding process. You certainly can't nurse the baby, but you can give bottle feedings to give your partner a break and give yourself added opportunities for closeness with your baby. If you have older children at home, spend extra time with them to help them get used to being big brothers or sisters.

Your caregiver will tell you when it's safe to resume sexual activity. Some couples are advised to wait up to six weeks postpartum. What you lose in sexual intercourse, you can make up by cuddling and massaging each other.

in a tub of warm water. You can also try putting peppermint oil in bath water to stimulate urination.

## Bowel Discomforts

Don't be surprised if you feel constipated following childbirth. You may not have a bowel movement for several days—usually because you don't need to. Mothers who are given meperidine for pain relief are especially likely to experience constipation. One way to keep your stools soft is to eat high-fiber foods, such as bran and fresh vegetables, and drink eight 8-ounce glasses of water every day. You will need the extra fluids for milk production while nursing, anyway.

### *Enemas*

Inserting a dab of olive oil in the rectum using a finger helps some women relieve constipation. Hospitals usually give collapsible enemas that soften the stool without pulling water from the bowels. Many caregivers give women laxatives such as castor oil to help them eliminate toxins and encourage breastfeeding. The usual dose is two ounces of cold press castor oil in an eight-ounce glass of orange juice.

## Breast Engorgement

The average mother produces enough breast milk for five babies, and this causes *breast engorgement*—painfully swollen, tender breasts and nipples. If engorgement develops, try breastfeeding first. If you don't breastfeed or find it too painful at first (because there are hard lumps or your breasts are hard), you'll need to empty your breasts yourself before *mastitis* (inflammation of the breast) sets in. You can empty your breasts by various methods, including breast pumps or hand expression methods. La Leche League counselors or your hospital's breastfeeding consultant can explain how.

Sage tea or capsules may help reduce engorgement. If your breasts are extra sensitive, make sure that the water does not touch them when you shower.

## Postpartum Depression

A small minority of women become depressed after giving birth. This is thought to be due to hormonal changes aggravated by a painful delivery, medical complications, or stress. The so-called "baby blues" generally begins the third or fourth day after the baby is born and is characterized by exhaustion, crying spells, and feelings of inadequacy. It usually disappears just as quickly as it appeared, especially if you revive your energy through exercise, massage, relaxation, diet, and vitamin and mineral supplements.

With your caregiver's guidance, try the holistic remedies for depression described in Chapter 2; i.e., aromatherapy (with jasmine, neroli, clary sage, or rose), botanical medicines (St. John's Wort supplements and chamomile or black walnut tea), guided imagery visualizations, massage, meditation, nutrition (high-protein foods, easy-to-digest vegetables and fruits, nuts, seeds, and beans), and vitamin and mineral supplements (vitamins C, $B_{12}$, $B_6$, $B_3$, folic acid, magnesium, and zinc).

If your depression lingers, call your caregiver immediately. In the worst scenario, you may need to take an antidepressant, in which case you won't be able to breastfeed because the chemicals are passed to the baby in your breast milk. Your caregiver may also recommend that you wear an estrogen patch. According to an article by Dr. John Studd that appeared in the September 1995 issue of *Lancet,* British doctors have helped relieve postpartum depression with skin patches that deliver estrogen into the bloodstream to boost serotonin levels. Black walnut supplements or tea also do this. According to Studd, estrogen patches don't suppress the milk production after breastfeeding has been established.

## Getting Back in Shape

Resuming your pregnancy exercise routine will not only help you get back into your former physical shape—it will also help you feel so much better because you know that you're doing something for yourself, rather than just waiting for healing to happen. Lack of sleep, nursing, and child care will place extra demands on your body. The fastest way to revive your energy is to resume safe, gentle exercises, such as Kegel exercises, swimming, walking, yoga, qigong, or tai chi.

If you had a normal vaginal birth, your caregiver may advise you to start a postpartum exercise program as early as 24 hours after delivery. If you had an episiotomy, your caregiver will probably recommend Kegel exercises, swimming, or walking. If you had a cesarean delivery, you'll have to wait about five weeks before your first postpartum workout, but you can do easy walking in the meantime.

Your hospital may have a postpartum exercise class, which could motivate you to get back into a fitness program as soon as possible. Most classes accept women whose bleeding has stopped and who can comfortably walk a half mile to a mile with no physical discomfort. Anytime your bleeding is pink or yellowish pink and then suddenly red, it's a sign that you're overdoing it and that you should go to bed with your baby and rest for twenty-four hours. If the bleeding does not stop, be sure to call your caregiver.

**Kegel Exercises**

You can start Kegel exercises the first day after giving birth while you're still in bed. You'll want to gently exercise your pelvic floor muscles and ligaments because they support the bladder, uterus, and rectum. For the first several days, focus on Kegel exercises, abdominal breathing exercises (pushing your belly out as you inhale and contracting your abdominals toward the spine on the exhale), and foot circles (rotating the feet in both directions) to increase your blood circulation and promote faster healing. Also, check with your caregiver about using the towel exercises described in Chapter 4 to get yourself back into shape.

**Yoga**

Yoga is the safest exercise that you can begin immediately after birth. It will help normalize your heart rate, blood pressure, and breathing, and gently exercise your pelvic and abdominal muscles so they do not become sore or tight. Practicing yoga will quickly and safely restore your aerobic fitness without raising your blood lactate levels, which causes muscle soreness. This, in turn, will give you more energy to nurse your baby. Yoga will also help you return to your pre-pregnancy body weight and shape faster.

**Weight Lifting**

By the third or fourth week after giving birth, you can start doing upper-body strengthening exercises without weights. Between four and six weeks after delivery, you may be able to add light weights (one to five pounds) with moderate repetitions of eight to twelve. You should take care, however, not to become fatigued. If you experience increased pelvic pain, discomfort, or bright red vaginal bleeding, reduce the intensity and duration of your exercise program and report your symptoms to your caregiver.

## Exercising with Your Baby

One of the biggest obstacles to exercising after childbirth is that you just don't want to be away from your baby. But the sooner you resume an active life, the better for both you and your baby. One thing you can do is go for walks, pushing the baby in a stroller. You can also try the following simple exercises that gently stretch your "mothering muscles," which include the upper, middle, and lower back; the pelvic region; and the arms, hips, abdominals, buttocks, and thighs.

1. While standing on level ground, place your left hand in the center of the stroller handle and your right hand on your hip. Stand to the right of the stroller, with your feet together.

2. Contract your abdominals, lift your torso, and tuck your buttocks under so that you feel as if your tailbone is pointing toward the ground.

3. Take a large step forward with your left foot, bending both knees so that your left knee is in line with your left ankle, your right knee points forward, and your right heel is off the ground.

4. At the same time, push the stroller forward, extending your left arm to chest height. Keep your torso lifted and abdominals contracted.

5. Straighten up, pushing off the back foot, and bringing the back foot forward so that your feet are together again. Be careful not to tip the stroller.

6. Repeat, stepping forward with the right foot.

Use the following exercise to strengthen your buttocks, lower back, and hamstrings.

1. Facing the stroller, put both hands on the handle. With your abdominals contracted and torso lifted, pull your right knee up toward your chest, rounding your back and keeping your left knee slightly bent for balance.

2. Push your right leg out behind you at hip height.

3. Contract your buttocks as you straighten your leg, then lower the leg to the ground.

4. Repeat, alternating with your left leg.

*Postpartum*
*Nutritional*
*Guidelines*

According to ACOG, following childbirth you should continue to follow the Basic Food Plan of whole-grains, vegetables, fruits, and milk and milk products (see Chapter 3). Try to consume at least three to four servings of calcium-rich foods each day. If for any reason you can't

---

## RETURNING TO WORK

In the United States, the customary time to return to work after a vaginal delivery is six weeks, and for a cesarean section, eight weeks. Some companies give longer paid maternity leaves; the Family Medical Leave Act (FMLA) allows twelve weeks unpaid. If there have been undue complications—such as infection, anemia, blood loss, or any other problems of delivery and recovery—your caregiver will indicate when you can return to work. Most companies will honor that recommendation.

---

tolerate low-fat milk, try low-fat cheese, yogurt, or fish with edible bones (such as salmon and sardines), and eat more dark green vegetables. If you don't satisfy your daily calcium requirements with alternatives to milk, take 600 milligrams of calcium supplements daily. Be sure to consume eight glasses of water daily, and ask your caregiver if you need to increase your consumption of other vitamins and minerals, especially iron and zinc. ACOG also advises taking vitamin D supplements if your diet is lacking in vitamin D-fortified foods and you have limited exposure to sunlight. Vegans (strict vegetarians who do not eat any animal products) will need to take supplements of vitamins D, $B_{12}$, iron, and zinc.

If you're breastfeeding, you'll need to consume more foods rich in protein, calcium, vitamin $B_{12}$, and magnesium. ACOG indicates that if you consume a minimum of 1,800 calories per day, and follow the Basic Meal Plan we described, you won't need to take vitamin and mineral supplements. You should discuss your postpartum food plan with your caregiver or with a breastfeeding counselor. Some women need to take iron, folate, vitamin $B_6$, calcium, zinc, or magnesium supplements if they are not consuming the RDAs by eating whole foods.

Here are other important ACOG nutritional recommendations for breastfeeding mothers:

▷ An alcohol intake of less than three drinks a day (one drink is equal to one-half ounce of alcohol—the equivalent of twelve ounces of beer, four ounces of wine, or one and one-fifth ounces of liquor) has not been shown to affect breastfeeding. More than three drinks, however, may make your child lethargic and interfere with your let-down reflex.

▷ Many midwives believe that the amount of caffeine in three cups of coffee a day can result in a hyperactive baby and decrease his or her ability to absorb iron.

▷ Smoking is bad for the mother's health and reduces her milk volume. Secondhand smoke is probably even worse for the baby.

▷ Prescription medicines may have an adverse impact on your baby. Always ask your caregiver about the safety of any medication before taking it.

▷ Dieting to lose weight is not advisable. You can expect to lose an average of two pounds a month following childbirth without affecting your milk volume. For obese women, a loss of four pounds a month is acceptable.

## Breastfeeding

We strongly recommend that you breastfeed, if at all possible. According to the La Leche League, there are very few women who cannot breastfeed. If your nipples are inverted, for example, you can wear small devices that can pull them out. If you want to return to work immediately, you can nurse early in the morning and in the evening, and supplement baby's feedings with formula. If, for any reason, you have difficulty breastfeeding, ask to see your hospital's lactation counselor or call La Leche League (1-800-368-4404) twenty-four hours a day and talk to a breastfeeding consultant.

## Breastfeeding Tips

1. Take three one-hour naps a day. During the first three days, it's essential that you get adequate rest. For the rest of the month, you should use your ingenuity to get into bed and take each of these naps.

2. Be patient. It may take two or three weeks to learn how to nurse and a couple of months to become an expert. Don't regard every mishap as a signal for panic. Don't become alarmed when your baby wants to nurse a lot—or not at all. Babies who suddenly nurse a lot more are not starving. They are going through a growth spurt—and their increased sucking increases your milk supply. Babies who are a little fussy at first are getting used to the new routine, just like Mom. In two to three days, you'll both start to develop a routine.

## BENEFITS OF BREASTFEEDING FOR YOUR BABY

Breastfeeding has many advantages for you and your baby which have been documented extensively in clinical trials. The most important benefits to your baby include the fact that it:

▷ Strengthens your baby's immune system by supplying lactoferrin, lysozymes, secretory immunoglobulins A, T, and B lymphocytes, and macrophages

▷ Increases the survival rate for low–birth-weight newborns

▷ Reduces the risk for gastrointestinal infections

▷ Protects against *necrotizing enterocolitis,* a serious intestinal disorder common in premature or low–birth-weight babies

▷ Increases the intelligence quotient (IQ)

▷ Enhances bonding between mother and baby

The benefits of breastfeeding for the mother include the fact that it:

▷ Stimulates contractions of the uterus and helps control postpartum blood loss

▷ Improves immune function

▷ Increases the mother's confidence in her parenting skills

▷ Helps the mother regain her pre-pregnancy weight (breastfeeding burns 500 to 2,000 calories daily)

3.  You can freeze excess breast milk, but don't use a microwave oven to reheat it—microwaves distribute heat unevenly and some of the liquid may be too hot for your baby. The radiation can also destroy substances in your breast milk that help protect your baby from infection. Instead, defrost the milk in your refrigerator or heat the milk container in warm water.

4.  Try a *mechanical lactation aid.* The simplest one is a nasal spray containing oxytocin, the "let-down" hormone. This is especially helpful for nervous mothers. If you decide to use it, you'll need a prescription from your caregiver.

5.  Drinking a cup of borage tea after meals and taking three brewer's yeast tablets daily can also stimulate let down.

**Conditioning the
Let-Down Reflex**

Sometimes a new mother's *let-down reflex* (response to normal stimulation for milk flow) doesn't work reliably, even after two or three months of nursing. If you have this problem, try the following suggestions to induce milk flow:

1.  Put the baby on a schedule, starting with his first feeding. Pick a reasonable time interval—say, every two hours—and feed him regularly. Don't let your baby sleep four or five hours while your milk production slows.

2.  If you have to miss a scheduled feeding, try expressing your milk manually to prevent engorgement.

3.  Take five minutes before feeding to sit down, put your feet up, close your eyes, and relax.

4.  Nurse in the same comfortable, quiet spot at each feeding. Take a drink of water before you nurse to stimulate your let-down reflex.

5.  Stimulate let down by rubbing your fingers quickly and lightly over your nipples until they tingle.

---

## HOW TO TELL IF YOUR BABY IS GETTING ENOUGH MILK

1.  If your baby has several bowel movements a day which are yellow. Babies who are not getting enough to eat have scanty stools which may be greenish in color.

2.  If the baby's diapers are wet. Ten wet diapers a day are an indication that the baby is receiving enough breast milk. If you're using disposal diapers, it's sometimes difficult to tell how wet they are. Use cloth diapers or let the baby lie naked on several old towels.

3.  If the baby is content with eight to eleven feedings per day, which is a normal, healthy nursing schedule. If you're nursing this often and have an adequate let down at each feeding, your baby should be getting enough milk.

4.  If your baby is gaining four to seven ounces a week.

5.  If the baby's stools are soft and fluffy. Some newborns have bowel movements only once a week after five weeks—but lots of wet diapers. This is normal. Breastfed babies do not become constipated because they absorb and utilize virtually all the breast milk without producing toxins—so they don't eliminate as much waste.

Many women find that they have less milk for their baby in the evening. If you've nursed the baby a lot during the day, your breasts may be empty at supper time. If you can't nurse at this time, keep baby occupied by giving him or her a massage. After a shower, a drink, and a good dinner, you should have ample milk to nurse until baby falls asleep.

When you first start nursing, you'll find that supply and demand fluctuate. It may take a couple of months for you and your baby to get synchronized, and even then there may be days when you have a little more or less milk than baby wants. Thus, a day of overfilling may be followed by a day of insufficiency and a day of skimpy milk supply, and constant nursing may well be followed by a day of super-abundance.

If your baby sleeps six, eight, or ten hours at night and you wake up every morning full of milk, try waking him or her in the middle of the night to nurse. In another month or two, both you and the baby will be able to go for longer periods of time between feedings. You can overcome night feeding problems by having the baby sleep in bed with you until you've nursed once, then put the baby back in his or her own bed.

## Baby Formulas

Breast milk is the best food for your baby—and it's free! Realistically, however, there will probably be times when you will need to give the baby some type of formula. Infant formulas are now available in ready-to-use, liquid concentrate, and powdered forms. Ready-to-use formulas offer the convenience of simply opening a can and pouring the liquid, but they're more expensive than the concentrate or powder. Concentrates and powdered formulas are relatively easy to prepare (you just add water), but be sure to follow the directions carefully so that the formula given to the baby is neither too strong nor too diluted.

If you feed your baby a cow's-milk–based formula and he or she develops frequent diarrhea, hives, a runny nose, or a rash, your baby may be allergic to cow's milk. In this case, a soy-based formula is a good substitute. If you suspect that your baby may have a problem with cow's milk, ask your caregiver or pediatrician if soy formula is a good alternative. Be aware that soy beverages, sometimes improperly called "soy milk," are not the same as soy-based infant formulas.

Unlike true infant formulas, which are nutritionally complete, soy beverages often lack several nutrients that infants need, including calcium and vitamins D, E, and C.

There are also formulas known as *protein hydrolysate* formulas, which don't cause allergic reactions because the proteins responsible for allergic reactions are already broken down. As with milk- and soy-based formulas, hydrolysate formulas are also available in powder, liquid concentrate, or ready-to-feed forms. Whatever form is chosen, proper preparation and refrigeration are essential. Opened cans of ready-to-feed and liquid concentrates should be properly stored and refrigerated and used within the time specified on the can. Once the powder is mixed with water, it should also be properly stored and refrigerated if it's not going to be used right away. Again, be sure to add the *exact* amount of water recommended on the label. Under-diluted formula can cause problems for the infant's organs and digestive system, and over-diluted formula will not provide adequate nutrition. Warming previously prepared formula isn't necessary if it has been stored properly, but a warm bottle is a lot friendlier and cozier, and some babies will refuse cold formula. Follow the manufacturer's recommendations regarding reheating the leftover formula in a bottle.

Make sure that your water source is pure (see Chapter 4). This is especially important if you're traveling out of the country with your baby and local water purity or refrigeration may be a problem.

# HOLISTIC APPROACHES TO COMMON BABY CARE

Jaundice

While babies are still inside the womb, they produce a lot of red blood cells. Several days after birth, their livers begin to break down the extra red blood cells, producing *bilirubin*. Bilirubin is excreted into the baby's skin and fat, and sometimes causes a yellowing of baby's skin and the whites of the eyes, a condition known as jaundice. Usually, jaundice appears during the second day after birth, peaks about the fourth day, and disappears by the sixth day. If your baby appears jaundiced, tell your caregiver or pediatrician. He or she may want to draw a blood sample to measure the bilirubin level in your baby's blood. If it's unusually high, you may be advised to keep your baby in the hospital for phototherapy for several days to lower the bilirubin levels.

It may be more effective, however, to expose your baby to natural sunlight, which research has shown works faster and with fewer side effects than phototherapy. Both natural and artificial phototherapy help eliminate bilirubin.

Jaundice that is present at birth or that develops within twenty-four hours after delivery is abnormal. It may be the result of infection, liver problems, or, more rarely, a blood type (ABO) incompatibility. Jaundice is particularly common in premature babies and can be dangerous. For example, bilirubin may be deposited in the brain—a condition known as *kernicterus*—which can lead to a lower IQ, cerebral palsy, or learning disabilities. This is a rare condition, however, which only occurs in preterm babies.

If your baby is full term, develops jaundice, but nurses well and seems healthy otherwise, you needn't worry. You should be able to take your baby home without resorting to phototherapy. You and your caregiver, however, should monitor your baby for possible signs of jaundice complications, such as lethargy, poor feeding, fever, pale-colored stools, dark urine, or frequent vomiting.

## Dry, Flaky Skin

Your newborn baby won't develop normal skin for several weeks, because it takes that long for their *sebaceous glands* to start secreting oil. The lack of this oil can result in dry, flaky skin. The best thing you can do is clean and massage your baby every day using baby oil made with purified water. When it's time to use shampoos, lotions, and powders, use only natural products, especially those containing calendula, chamomile, aloe, and vitamins E and A.

Some baby skin moisturizers contain olive oil, which is excellent for removing cradle cap—the dry, flaky scalp seen on some babies. Rub the olive oil gently into your baby's scalp; if your baby has hair, comb the oil through with a fine-tooth comb.

## Diaper Rash

Many newborns develop diaper rash. You can avoid it by wiping the rash with a mixture of one ounce distilled white vinegar and six ounces of water. Wiping the baby with a cream ointment of calendula or comfrey also works. Talc sometimes aggravates the skin; use baby powders with rose, slippery elm bark, or myrrh instead. Cornstarch or cornstarch plus baking soda is also good.

Be very careful about exposing your newborn to the sun. Ask your pediatrician how much you can expose the baby to sunlight and what types of sunscreens are safe.

## Colic and Crying

Excessive crying which lasts more than three weeks is usually considered colic. Normal babies cry a lot, so you shouldn't assume that just because your infant is irritable for more than three hours a day that something is wrong. More than likely, it's just your baby's way of letting you know that he or she is healthy, energetic, and alive. Studies show that most colicky babies stop crying at the end of three months.

Although pediatricians don't know exactly what causes colic, here are several tips for dealing with it:

▷ *Let your baby sleep.* To determine whether your child is crying because of fatigue, try feeding, burping, changing, or cuddling first. If the baby is still crying, put him or her down to sleep, and walk away. Some babies do not like to be held to sleep.

▷ *Stay calm.* Colic has never been known to cause any serious medical problems. By staying calm, you tell the baby that he or she has your attention, but that his crying will have to end soon.

▷ *Avoid cow's milk.* The protein in cow's milk is hard for most newborns to digest properly. It enters the baby's bloodstream and triggers an allergic response. This can be very uncomfortable for baby, making him or her seem "colicky." The protein may be responsible for colic in 5 to 10 percent of babies who suffer from the condition. Use commercial baby formula (in which the protein is partially digested) or try a soy-based formula. If your baby's crying does not improve after five days, you can assume that milk is not the problem.

▷ *Peppermint water.* Peppermint-flavored water can help relax the baby's intestines. You can soak peppermint leaf in water, and then feed a bottle full of the flavored water to your baby. Undiluted peppermint oil is too strong for the baby and should never be used without water. Giving baby a cooled tea made of one-half teaspoon of powdered fennel or anise leaves added to a cup of boiling water will also help.

Teething

When a several-months-old infant suddenly becomes fussier than usual, the baby is probably cutting a tooth. Teething babies typically need to "work" their gums, and do so by chewing on crib edges, teething rings, bottle nipples, their parents' fingers, or their own fingers. The baby may also have looser stools than usual. Teething (or cutting even one tooth) can take several weeks, and the irritability and loose stools will come and go.

---

## PREVENTING POTENTIAL PROBLEMS

Chances are your baby will be perfectly healthy. But there are some potential problems you need to be aware of.

▷ **Respiratory disorders.** The majority of first-year infant deaths involve respiratory disorders—an infant's inability to breathe naturally. Many premature babies are born without *surfactant,* the liquid that coats the inside of the air sacs in the lungs to keep them from collapsing when they exhale. Most preemies are put on a respirator or other mechanical device until their lungs mature and produce their own surfactant. Until they produce their own surfactant, they are usually given Exosurf®—a white, foamy liquid drug that has proven successful in treating many infant respiratory disorders. It's administered by inserting a tube down an infant's airway soon after birth and spraying the mist into its lungs. Some babies show immediate improvement.

▷ **Low–birth-weight baby.** The second most common cause of infant mortality is low birth weight—babies who weigh five and a half pounds or less at birth. These babies are forty times more likely to die within the first four weeks of life. If they survive, low–birth-weight babies are far more likely to have a permanent disability. Premature babies and infants born to substance-abusing mothers are at high risk for being born with low birth weights and with disabilities.

▷ **Sudden Infant Death Syndrome (SIDS).** Every year one to two per thousand live births result in SIDS; overall, 6,000 to 8,000 babies die of SIDS each year. The peak age for death from SIDS is two to four months, and more deaths occur in winter than other times of the year. Babies who sleep on their stomachs have the highest rate of SIDS. The American Academy of Pediatrics now recommends that babies sleep on their backs to help prevent the fatal disorder. Be sure your baby sleeps on a flat, firm mattress without any plush bedding. No soft, fluffy products such as pillows, sheepskins, or toys should be placed under baby's mouth while sleeping. We recommend that you have your baby sleep with you on his or her back with their face towards you so you can monitor them periodically during the night.

One safe way of relieving teething pain is to give your baby a pacifier which contains crushed ice, or a bottle containing a few ounces of cold water which will cool baby's gums. If the baby continues to be irritated, he may have a gum infection, so check with your pediatrician.

# $\mathcal{A}$ FINAL WORD

Your journey of holistic pregnancy and childbirth has come to an end. Along the way we introduced you to many holistic remedies from many different cultures. We walked, so to speak, with two feet on the ground, recommending the safest, most effective approaches of both modern and traditional medicine.

In closing, we leave you and your baby with a prayer affirmation which many Canadian midwives give newborn mothers.

*Nature is my mother.*

*The universe is my way.*

*Eternity is my kingdom.*

*Mind is my home.*

*Truth is my workshop.*

*Love is my law.*

*Conscience is my guide.*

*Peace is my shelter.*

*Experience is my school.*

*Obstacle is my lesson.*

*Difficulty is my stimulant.*

*Joy is my hymn.*

*Pain is my warning.*

*Light is my realization.*

*Friend is my companion.*

*Adversity is my instructor.*

*Neighbor is my brother.*

*Struggle is my opportunity.*

*Future time is my promise.*

*Equilibrium is my attitude.*

*Order is my path.*

*Beauty is my ideal.*

*Perfection is my destiny.*

You have created a human life, the most important work on this planet, and we sincerely thank you for letting us travel with you.

James Marti
*Executive Director, Holistic Medical Research Foundation*

Heather Burton
*Licensed Midwife, Founder of the Midwives Alliance*

# $\mathcal{A}$PPENDIX A: MONTHLY CHECKUP FORMS

Holistic Pregnancy Program
Monthly Checkup Forms
*(We recommend that you and your caregiver complete
these forms during your monthly checkups.)*

## FIRST-MONTH CHECKUP

Date _____

Weeks pregnant _____

Weight _____

Blood pressure _____

Protein/sugar levels _____

Fetal heart rate _____

Fundal height _____

Presentation _____

## Holistic Therapies Recommended by Caregiver

Fatigue_____

Frequent urination_____

Nausea_____

Vomiting _____

Morning sickness_____

Excessive salivation (pytalism)_____

Heartburn _____

Indigestion _____

— ▲ —

## SECOND-MONTH CHECKUP

Date _____

Weeks pregnant _____

Weight _____

Blood pressure _____

Protein/sugar levels _____

Fetal heart rate _____

Fundal height _____

Presentation _____

## Holistic Therapies Recommended by Caregiver

Flatulence _____

Constipation _____

Food cravings _____

Sweating _____

— ▲ —

## THIRD-MONTH CHECKUP

Date _____

Weeks pregnant _____

Weight _____

Blood pressure _____

Protein/sugar levels _____

Fetal heart rate _____

Fundal height _____

Presentation _____

## Holistic Therapies Recommended by Caregiver

Tension headaches _____

Digestive headaches _____

Migraines_____

Neck pains _____

Fainting _____

Dizziness_____

Bloating_____

— ▲ —

# FOURTH-MONTH CHECKUP

Date _____

Weeks pregnant _____

Weight _____

Blood pressure _____

Protein/sugar levels _____

Fetal heart rate _____

Fundal height _____

Presentation _____

## Holistic Therapies Recommended by Caregiver

Corpus luteum cysts _____

Hemorrhoids_____

Vaginal discharge (leukorrhea) _____

Nasal congestion _____

Nosebleeds _____

— ▲ —

# FIFTH-MONTH CHECKUP

Date _____

Weeks pregnant _____

Weight _____

Blood pressure _____

*(Fifth-Month Checkup continued)*

Protein/sugar levels _____

Fetal heart rate _____

Fundal height _____

Presentation _____

## Holistic Therapies Recommended by Caregiver

Herpes_____

Menstrual-like cramps_____

Skin rashes _____

Stretch marks_____

Moderately high blood pressure_____

Pregnancy-induced hypertension (PIH)_____

Edema _____

Insomnia _____

— ▲ —

# SIXTH-MONTH CHECKUP

Date _____

Weeks pregnant _____

Weight _____

Blood pressure _____

Protein/sugar levels _____

Fetal heart rate _____

Fundal height _____

Presentation _____

## Holistic Therapies Recommended by Caregiver

Hemorrhoids_____

Vaginal discharge (leukorrhea) _____

Leg cramps _____

Backaches_____

Varicose veins_____

— ▲ —

## SEVENTH-MONTH CHECKUP

Date _____

Weeks pregnant _____

Weight _____

Blood pressure _____

Protein/sugar levels _____

Fetal heart rate _____

Fundal height _____

Presentation _____

## Holistic Therapies Recommended by Caregiver

Lower abdominal pain _____

Changes in skin pigmentation _____

Fatigue _____

Shortness of breath _____

Overheating _____

Inadequate weight gain _____

— ▲ —

## EIGHTH-MONTH CHECKUP

Date _____

Weeks pregnant _____

Weight _____

Blood pressure _____

Protein/sugar levels _____

Fetal heart rate _____

Fundal height _____

Presentation _____

## Holistic Therapies Recommended by Caregiver

Incompetent cervix _____

*(Eighth-Month Checkup continued)*

Uterine irritability_____

Placenta previa (low-lying placenta)_____

Sciatica_____

Fetal hiccups_____

Overheating _____

Leaking of colostrum_____

— ▲ —

# Ninth-Month Checkups (Include each visit)

Date_____

Weeks pregnant _____

Weight_____

Blood pressure _____

Protein/sugar levels _____

Fetal heart rate _____

Fundal height _____

Presentation _____

Internal cervix examination _____

## Holistic Therapies Recommended by Caregiver

Chronic backaches_____

Frequent urination after the baby drops_____

Prelabor symptoms _____

Back labor_____

Irregular contractions _____

— ▲ —

Date_____

Weeks pregnant _____

Weight_____

Blood pressure _____

Protein/sugar levels _____

Fetal heart rate _____

Fundal height _____

Presentation _____

Internal cervix examination _____

## Holistic Therapies Recommended by Caregiver

Chronic backaches _____

Frequent urination after the baby drops_____

Prelabor symptoms _____

Back labor_____

Irregular contractions_____

—— ▲ ——

Date_____

Weeks pregnant _____

Weight _____

Blood pressure _____

Protein/sugar levels _____

Fetal heart rate _____

Fundal height _____

Presentation _____

Internal cervix examination _____

## Holistic Therapies Recommended by Caregiver

Chronic backaches_____

Frequent urination after the baby drops_____

Prelabor symptoms _____

Back labor_____

Irregular contractions_____

—— ▲ ——

# POSTPARTUM CHECKUP

Date _____

Weight _____

Blood pressure _____

Uterine examination _____

Breast examination _____

## Holistic Therapies Recommended by Caregiver for Mother

Afterpains _____

Fatigue_____

Fever _____

Perineal pain_____

Incisional pain _____

Bowel discomfort_____

Constipation _____

Exhaustion _____

Depression _____

Difficulty urinating_____

Breast engorgement_____

Difficulty breastfeeding_____

## Postpartum Checkup of Baby

General appearance: _____

Skin _____

Eyes_____

Ears _____

Nose_____

Mouth _____

Neck _____

Heart _____

Lungs_____

Abdomen_____

Arms and legs_____

Hips _____

Pulse _____

Neurologic_____

## Holistic Therapies Recommended by Caregiver for Baby

Jaundice_____

Dry, flaky skin _____

Diaper rash _____

Colic and crying_____

— ▲ —

# $\mathcal{A}$PPENDIX B: REFERENCES

## CHAPTER 1

Altman, Nathaniel. *Everybody's Guide to Chiropractic Health Care.* Los Angeles: Jeremy P. Tarcher, Inc., 1989.

Boyle, Wade. *Lectures in Naturopathic Hydrotherapy.* East Palestine, Ohio: Buckeye Naturopathic Press, 1988.

Cerney, James. *Acupuncture Without Needles.* New York: Parker Publishing Co., 1983.

Chopra, Deepak. *Perfect Health: The Complete Mind/Body Guide.* New York: Harmony Books, 1995.

Chopra, Deepak. *Quantum Healing.* New York: Bantam Publishing, 1991.

Edell, Dean. "Medical Journal." *San Jose Mercury News.* (July 22, 1993): 9.

Epstein, Gerald. *Healing Visualizations.* New York: Bantam Books, 1989.

Goleman, Daniel. *The Meditative Mind.* Los Angeles: Jeremy P. Tarcher, 1988.

Green, Elmer, and Green, Alyce. *Beyond Biofeedback.* New York: McGraw-Hill, 1991.

Hahnemann, Samuel. *Organon of Medicine.* Translated by W. Boericke, M.D. New Delhi: B. Jain Publishers, 1992.

Hochstrasser, Bernard. "Homeopathy And Conventional Medicine in the Management of Pregnancy and Childbirth." *Homeopathic Education Services,* January 1994; 1–4.

Jain, Steven. "A Study of Response Pattern of Non-Insulin Dependent Diabetics To Yoga Therapy." *Diabetes Research & Clinical Practice.* (January 1993): 69–74.

Labrecque, Michael. "Prevention of Perineal Trauma by Perineal Massage during Pregnancy." *Birth.* (March 1994): 20–25.

Lavarbre, Marcel. *Aromatherapy Workbook.* Berkeley, California: Healing Arts Press, 1991.

Porkett, Manfred. *Chinese Medicine.* New York: Henry Holt & Co, 1992.

Siegel, Bernie. *Love, Medicine & Miracles.* New York: Harper & Row, 1986.

Siegel, Bernie. *Peace, Love and Healing.* New York: Harper Perennial, 1991.

The Burton Goldberg Group. *Alternative Medicine: The Definitive Guide.* Payallup, Wash.: Future Medicine Publishing, 1993.

Tirtha, Swami Shiva. "Ayurveda and Childbirth." *Ayurveda Journal.* (March 1997): 4.

Vishnu-devananda, Swami. *The Complete Book of Yoga.* New York: Harmony Books, 1988.

## CHAPTER 2

"Appetite for Life." *Fit Pregnancy.* (Summer 1996): 52.

Balch, James F., and Balch, Phyllis. *Prescription for Nutritional Healing.* Garden City Park, N.Y.: Avery Publishing, 1993.

Beinfield, Harriet. *Between Heaven and Earth: A Guide to Chinese Medicine.* New York: Ballantine Books, 1991.

Bellumini, James. "Acupressure For Nausea and Vomiting of Pregnancy: A Randomized, Blinded Study." *Obstetrics & Gynecology* (August 1994): 245–48.

Bennings, Michael. "Biofeedback Training in Chronic Constipation." *Archives of Disease.* (January 1993): 126–29.

Blatt, Robin J. *Prenatal Tests: What They Are, Their Benefits and Risks, and How to Decide Whether to Have Them or Not.* New York: Vintage Press, 1988.

Charlish, Anne. *Birth-Tech: Tests and Technology in Pregnancy and Birth.* New York: Facts on File, 1990.

Cummings, Stephen, and Ullman, Dana. *Everybody's Guide to Homeopathic Medicine.* New York: St. Martin's Press, 1991.

Erick, Miriam. *No More Morning Sickness: A Survival Guide for Pregnant Women.* New York: Plume, 1993.

Gach, Michael. *Acupressure's Potent Points: A Guide to Self-Care for Common Ailments.* New York: Bantam Books, 1993.

Hoffman, David. *The New Holistic Herbal.* Rockport, Mass.: Element Books, 1992.

Institute of Medicine. "Nutrition During Pregnancy." *Weight Gain and Nutrient Supplements.* Washington, D.C.: National Academy Press, 1990.

Morales, Karla, and Inlander, Charles B. *Take This Book to the Obstetrician with You.* New York: Addison-Wesley, 1991.

National Center For Health Statistics. "Number of In-Hospital Midwife Attended Births." *Monthly Vital Statistics Report.* (February 1993).

Resnick, Susan Kushner. "My Baby: Childbirth That Blends Tradition and Technology." *Natural Health.* (November/December, 1993): 86–87.

Rooks, James. "Outcomes of Care in Birth Centers." *New England Journal of Medicine* (August 1989): 1804.

Ryman, Daniele. *Aromatherapy: The Encyclopedia of Plants and Oils and How They Help You.* New York: Bantam Books, 1993.

Scott, Aurelia. "Midwives Deliver." *Country Journal.* (January–February, 1995): 12–15.

Taxel, Laura. "Doulas Help Deliver Healthy Babies." *Natural Health* (July/August 1993): 44–48.

U.S. Food and Drug Administration. "Caffeine Content of Food and Beverages." *Healthy Eating During Pregnancy.* White Plains, N.Y.: March of Dimes Birth Defects Foundation, 1993.

Worsley, J. R. *Acupuncture: Is It for You?* New York: Harper & Row, 1973.

## CHAPTER 3

"Folate Deficiency And Pregnancy Outcome." *Nutrition Review,* (October 1991): 314–15.

"Healthy Eating During Pregnancy." International Food Information Council Foundation. White Plains, N.Y., 1997.

Abrams, Richard. *Will It Hurt The Baby? The Safe Use of Medications during Pregnancy and Breast-Feeding.* New York: Addison-Wesley Publishing Co, 1990.

American College of Obstetricians and Gynecologists (ACOG). "Nutrition During Pregnancy." *ACOG Technical Bulletin.* Washington, D.C.: February 1994.

American College of Obstetricians and Gynecologists (ACOG). "Screening For Drug Abuse." *ACOG Technical Bulletin.* Washington, D.C.: December 1997.

Briggs, Gerald et al. *Drugs in Pregnancy and Lactation: A Reference Guide to Fetal and Neonatal Risk.* Baltimore: Williams & Wilkins, 1994.

Food and Nutrition Board, Institute of Medicine, National Academy of Sciences, *Nutrition during Pregnancy. Part 1: Weight Gain; Part 2: Nutrient Supplements.* Washington, D.C.: National Academy Press, 1990.

Forest, Franz. "Reported Social Alcohol Consumption During Pregnancy and Infant's Development at 18 Months." *British Medical Journal.* (July 6, 1991): 22–26.

Glenn, Foster. "Fluoride Tablet Supplementation during Pregnancy for Caries Immunity." *American Journal of Obstetrics & Gynecology.* (April 1982): 560.

Knight, Karl. "Calcium Supplementation In Normotensive and Hypertensive Pregnant Women." *American Journal of Clinical Nutrition.* (May 1992): 891–95.

Krishna, Raul. "Transfer of Cocaine by the Perfused Human Placenta: The Effect of Binding to Serum Proteins." *American Journal Of Obstetrics & Gynecology.* (December 1993): 1418–23.

Marya, Ronald. "Effect of Vitamin D Supplementation during Pregnancy on the Neonatal Skeletal Growth." *Annals Of Nutrition & Metabolism.* (December 1991): 208–12.

Mead, Nathaniel. "Pregnant? Get Your Vitamin D." *Natural Health.* (January/February 1995): 18.

National Research Council, National Academy of Sciences. *Nutrition during Pregnancy.* Washington, D.C.: National Academy Press, 1990.

National Research Council, National Academy of Sciences. *Recommended Dietary Allowances,* 10th ed., 1989.

Olsen, Frank. "Randomized Control Trial of Effect of Fish-Oil Supplementation on Pregnancy Duration." *Lancet* (April 1992): 1003–7.

Popeski, Daniel. "Blood Pressure during Pregnancy in Canadian Inuit: Community Differences Related to Diet." *Canadian Medical Association Journal.* (September 1, 1991): 445–54.

Sanders, Thomas. "Vegetarian Diets and Children." *American Journal of Clinical Nutrition.* (May 1994):1176–81.

Scholl, Tracy. "Anemia versus Iron Deficiency: Increased Risk of Preterm Delivery in a Prospective Study." *American Journal of Clinical Nutrition.* (May 1992): 985–88.

Somer, Elizabeth. *Nutrition for Women: The Complete Guide.* New York: Henry Holt Publishers, 1994.

Springer, Eileen. "Caffeine And Pregnancy." *American Health.* (September 1993): 86.

Taper, Lawrence. "Zinc and Copper Retention during Pregnancy: The Adequacy of Prenatal Diets with and without Dietary Supplementation." *American Journal of Clinical Nutrition.* (August 1985): 1184–92.

# CHAPTER 4

American College of Obstetricians and Gynecologists. "Exercise during Pregnancy and the Postpartum Period." *Technical Bulletin.* Washington, D.C.: 1994.

"Exercise During Pregnancy." *Health Tips Index.* (June 1990): 1–2.

"Headache." *Mayo Clinic Health Letter* (October 1993):1–8.

Artal, Raul. *Pregnancy and Exercise.* New York: Delacorte, 1992.

Chaitow, Leon. *The Body/Mind Purification Program.* New York: Simon & Schuster, 1990.

Jordan, Sandra. *Yoga for Pregnancy.* New York: St. Martin's Press, 1987.

Olkin, Sylvia. *Positive Pregnancy Fitness: A Guide to a More Comfortable Pregnancy and Easier Birth Through Exercise and Relaxation.* Garden City Park, N.Y.: Avery Publishing Group, 1993.

Schatz, Mary. *A Doctor's Gentle Yoga Program for Back and Neck Pain Relief.* Berkeley, Calif.: Rodmell Publishers, 1992.

# CHAPTER 5

"Indoor Air Pollution." *Mayo Clinic Health Letter.* (November 1993): 6.

"Two-thirds of the U.S. Population Breathes Polluted Air." *Natural Health.* (September/October 1993): 12–13.

Agency for Toxic Substance and Disease Registry. *The Nature and Extent of Lead Poisoning in the United States.* Washington, D.C.: Agency for Toxic Substance and Disease Registry, 1988.

Benson, Herbert. *Beyond the Relaxation Response.* New York: Berkeley Books, 1985.

Borysenko, Joan. *Minding the Body, Mending the Mind.* New York: Bantam Books, 1987.

Chopra, Deepak. *Quantum Healing.* New York: Crown Publishers, 1994.

Cook, Judith. *Dirty Water.* London: Unwin Hyman, 1989.

Dudley, Nigel. *The Poisoned Earth.* London: Piatkus Publishers, 1987.

Environmental Protection Agency. Office of Air and Radiation. *The Inside Story: A Guide to Indoor Air Quality.* Washington, D.C.: Office of Air and Radiation, Environmental Protection Agency, September 1988.

Greeley, Alexandra. "Getting the Lead Out of Just About Everything." *FDA Consumer Reports.* (July/August) 1991: 26–31.

Haddy, Ronald. "Aging, Infections, and the Immune System." *Journal of Family Practice.* (October 1988): 409–13.

Hilts, Peter. "Studies Say Soot Kills Up to 60,000 in U.S. Each Year." *New York Times.* (July 19, 1993): 7.

LeShan, Lawrence. *How to Meditate.* New York: Bantam Books, 1974.

Marwick, Charles. "Immune System Yields Its Secrets." *New England Journal of Medicine.* (November 24, 1989): 2786–87.

Nossal, Gerald. "The Basic Components of the Immune System." *New England Journal of Medicine.* (May 21, 1989): 1320–25.

Popeski, Daniel. "Blood Pressure during Pregnancy in Canadian Inuit: Community Differences Related To Diet." *Canadian Medical Association Journal.* (September 1, 1991): 445–54.

Schecter, Steven. *Fighting Radiation and Chemical Pollutants with Foods, Herbs and Vitamins.* Berkeley, Calif.: Vitality, 1990.

Wedeen, Ronald. *Poison in the Pot: The Legacy of Lead.* Carbondale, Ill.: Southern Illinois University Press, 1984.

# CHAPTER 6

"Hypertension: Lower Your Blood Pressure without Drugs." *Mayo Clinic Health Letter.* (May 1990): 2–3.

Altman, Nathaniel. *Oxygen Healing Therapies.* New York: Health Sciences Press, 1994.

American Heart Association. *About High Blood Pressure.* Dallas: American Heart Association, 1986.

Davis, Julie. *Young Skin for Life.* Emmaus, Penn.: Rodale Press, 1995.

Dawson, Eric. "Magnesium and Lead Relationships In Pre-eclampsia." *American Journal of Clinical Nutrition.* (May 1990): 512.

Eliasson, Karl. "A Dietary Fiber Supplement in the Treatment of Mild Hypertension." *Journal of Hypertension.* (February 1992): 195–99.

Epstein, Ernst. *Common Skin Disorders,* 4th ed. New York: W. B. Saunders & Co., 1994.

Hamiltion, Richard. *The Herpes Handbook.* Portland: VDAC Press, 1997.

Hamilton, Richard. *The Herpes Book.* Portland: VDAC Press, 1996.

Homuth, Victor. "Clinical Aspects and Differential Therapy of Mild Hypertension in Pregnancy." *Gynecology Journal.* (May 1994): 267–70.

Jin, Paul. "Efficacy of Tai Chi, Brisk Walking, Meditation and Reading in Reducing Mental and Emotional Stress." *Journal of Psychosomatic Research.* (May 1992): 61–70.

Medical Help International, Inc. *Herpes.* Melbourne, Fla.: Medical Help International, 1997.

Moser, Marvin. *Lower Your Blood Pressure and Live Longer.* New York: Random House, 1989.

National High Blood Pressure Information Center. *High Blood Pressure and What You Can Do About It.* Bethesda: National High Blood Pressure Information Center, 1987.

Ornish, Dean. *Dr. Dean Ornish's Program for Reversing Heart Disease.* New York: Ballantine Books, 1990.

Steinberg, Philip. "Cat's Claw Update." *Townsend Letter for Doctors.* (August/September, 1995): 70–72.

Werbach, Melvyn. "Nutritional Influence on Illness: Toxemia of Pregnancy." *Townsend Letter for Doctors.* (July 1994): 714.

## CHAPTER 7

Altman, Nathaniel. *Everybody's Guide to Chiropractic Health Care.* Los Angeles: Jeremy P. Tarcher, 1989.

Cummings, Stephen, and Dana Ullman. *Everybody's Guide to Homeopathic Medicine.* New York: St. Martin's Press, 1991.

Diakow, Paul. "Back Pain During Pregnancy And Labor." *Journal of Manipulative & Physiological Therapeutics.* (February 1991): 116–18.

Dick-Read, Grantly. *Childbirth Without Fear.* Revised by Harlan E. Ellis. New York: Harper & Row Publishers, 1984.

Olkin, Sylvia. *Positive Pregnancy Fitness: A Guide to a More Comfortable Pregnancy and Easier Birth Through Exercise and Relaxation.* Garden City Park, N.Y.: Avery Publishing Group, 1993.

Schatz, Mary. *Back Care Basics: A Doctor's Gentle Yoga Program for Back and Neck Pain Relief.* Berkeley, Calif.: Rodmell Press, 1992.

## CHAPTER 8

"Healthy Eating during Pregnancy." International Food Information Council Foundation and March of Dimes Birth Defects Foundation, Community Services Division. White Plains, New York: 1997.

Abrams, Richard. *Will It Hurt the Baby? The Safe Use of Medications during Pregnancy and Breast-feeding.* New York: Addison-Wesley, 1990.

American College of Obstetricians and Gynecologists (ACOG). "Nutrition During Pregnancy." *ACOG Technical Bulletin.* Washington, D.C.: ACOG, February 1994.

Artal, Raul. *Pregnancy and Exercise.* New York: Delacorte, 1992.

Food and Nutrition Board, Institute of Medicine, National Academy of Sciences, *Nutrition During Pregnancy. Part 1: Weight Gain; Part 2: Nutrient Supplements.* Washington, D.C.: National Academy Press, 1990.

National Research Council, National Academy of Sciences. *Recommended Dietary Allowances,* 10th ed., 1989.

## CHAPTER 9

American College of Obstetricians and Gynecologists (ACOG). "Cesarean Births." *ACOG Technical Bulletin.* Washington, DC: ACOG, February 1994.

Jones, Charles. *Birth Without Surgery: A Guide to Preventing Unnecessary Cesareans.* New York: Dodd, Mead, 1987.

Mitchel, Karl. *Cesarean Birth: A Couple's Guide for Decision and Preparation.* New York: Beaufort Books, 1985.

Olsen, Frank. "Randomized Control Trial of Effect of Fish-Oil Supplementation on Pregnancy Duration." *Lancet.* (April 27, 1992): 1003–7.

Richards, Laurie. *When Pregnancy Isn't Perfect: A Layperson's Guide to Complications in Pregnancy* New York: Dutton, 1991.

Rich, Laurie. *The Vaginal Birth after Cesarean Experience.* South Hadley, Mass.: Bergin & Garvey, 1987.

## CHAPTER 10

Bergman, Rhonda. "The Birth Place." *Hospitals & Health Networks.* (December 5, 1994): 11–13.

Dick-Read, Grantly. *Childbirth without Fear.* Revised by Harlan E. Ellis. New York: Harper & Row Publishers, 1984.

Letts, Pamela J. "Smooth Delivery: Use Your Brain to Control Pain." *Journal of Women's Health.* (Winter 1993): 12–15.

Munson, Marty. "Hypnosis." *Prevention.* (June 1994): 38–43.

Oberg, Oscar. "Reflex Analgesia (Acupuncture) in the Treatment of Pregnant Women." *Akusherstyo i Ginekologiaa* (Russian). (February 1991): 37–39.

Olkin, Sylvia. *Positive Pregnancy Fitness: A Guide to a More Comfortable Pregnancy and Easier Birth Through Exercise and Relaxation.* Garden City Park, N.Y.: Avery Publishing Group, 1993.

Rich, Laurie. *When Pregnancy Isn't Perfect: A Layperson's Guide to Complications in Pregnancy.* New York: Dutton, 1991.

Wathen, Phillip. "Abnormal Uterine Bleeding During Labor." *Medical Clinics of North America.* (March 1995): 329–44.

# CHAPTER 11

"Touch: Don't Underestimate the Power of a Caring Hand." *Mayo Clinic Health Letter.* (June 1994): 7.

Benson, Michael. *Birth Day! The Last 24 Hours of Pregnancy.* Paragon Press, 1993.

Labrecque, Michael. "Prevention of Perineal Trauma by Perineal Massage during Pregnancy." *Birth.* (March 1994): 20–25.

Munson, Marty. "Smooth Delivery: Use Your Brain to Control Pain." *Prevention.* (June, 1994): 38.

Schneider, Virginia. *Infant Massage: A Handbook for Loving Parents.* New York: Bantam Books, 1994.

# CHAPTER 12

"Breast-feeding Helps Reduce Ear Infections for Baby." *Your Health.* (January 1994): 54.

"Exercise during Pregnancy and the Postpartum Period." American College of Obstetricians and Gynecologists. *ACOG Technical Bulletin.* Washington, D.C.: ACOG, February 1994.

"Nursing Mothers Lose More Fat After Birth." *Health & Fitness.* (September 1993): 13.

"Sleeping with Mom Safer for Babies." *Medical Tribune News.* (June 8, 1994): 11.

Food and Nutrition Board, Institute of Medicine, National Academy of Sciences. *Nutrition During Pregnancy. Part 2: Postpartum.* Washington, D.C.: National Academy Press, 1990.

La Leche League. *The Womanly Art of Breastfeeding.* Schaumburg, Ill.: La Leche League, 1992.

Lucas, Arnold. "Breast Milk and Subsequent Intelligence Quotient in Children." *Lancet.* (February 1992): 261–62.

Food and Nutrition Board, Institute Of Medicine, National Academy Of Sciences. *Nutrition During Pregnancy.* Washington, D.C.: National Academy Press, 1990.

National SIDS Foundation. *Facts about SIDS.* (July 1989): 1–3.

"New Drug Reducing Infant Mortality." *San Jose Mercury News.* (May 2, 1991): 7.

"Preventing Sudden Infant Death Syndrome." *Natural Health.* (September/October 1993): 64.

Public Health Service. Sudden Infant Death Syndrome Program. *Fact Sheet: What is SIDS?* (1994): 1–2.

Salmon, Margaret. *Breast Milk—Nature's Perfect Formula.* Demarest, N.J.: Techkits, 1997.

Studd, John. "Estrogen Patches and Postpartum Depression." *Lancet.* (September 1995): 1231–35.

"Sugar-Coated Infant Care a Sweet Success." *Tufts University Diet & Nutrition Newsletter.* (November 1994): 12.

# APPENDIX C: SOURCES FOR MORE INFORMATION

## CHAPTER 1

### Organizations

American Association of Naturopathic Physicians. 2366 Eastlake Avenue, Suite 322, Seattle, Washington 98102.

American College of Obstetricians and Gynecologists (ACOG) Resource Center. 409 12th Street S.W., Washington, D.C. 20024. For information on pregnancy and women's health, enclose a stamped, self-addressed envelope along with the subject of your request.

American Holistic Medical Association. 4101 Lake Boone Trail, Suite 201, Raleigh, North Carolina 27607.

Healthy Mother, Healthy Baby Coalition. Distributes helpful pamplets on pregnancy safety and childbirth. 409 12th Street SW, Washington, D.C. (800) 424-8576

International Childbirth Education Association. P.O. Box 20048, Minneapolis, MN 55420.

March of Dimes Birth Defects Foundation Community Services Division. Provides information on many pregnancy and childbirth subjects, especially prenatal hazards. 1275 Mamaroneck Avenue, White Plains, N.Y. 10705. (914) 428-7100.

Maternal and Child Health Center. Provides information to both the public and professionals on pregnancy and childbirth. (202) 625-8410

National Women's Health Network. 1325 G Street N.W., Washington, D.C. 20005.

Planned Parenthood Foundation of America. 810 Seventh Avenue, New York, N.Y. 10014.

### Recommended Reading

Bellumini, Jon. "Acupressure for Nausea and Vomiting of Pregnancy: A Randomized, Blinded Study." *Obstetrics & Gynecology* (August 1994): 245–48.

Berger, Bernard. "Mood Alteration with Yoga and Swimming: Aerobic Exercise May Not Be Necessary." *Perceptual & Motor Skills.* (December 1992): 1331–43.

Cardini, Frank. "Moxibustion and Breech Presentation. *American Journal of Chinese Medicine.* (August 1991): 105–14.

De Aloysia, Donald. "Morning Sickness Control in Early Pregnancy by Neiguan Point Acupressure." *Obstetrics & Gynecology.* (November 1992): 852–54.

Gach, Michael. *Acupressure's Potent Points: A Guide to Self-Care for Common Ailments.* New York: Bantam Books, 1993.

Gerhard, Irwin. "Auricular Acupuncture in the Treatment of Female Infertility." *Gynecological Endocrinology.* (September 1992): 171–81.

Graf, Frank. "Nongenetic Perinatal Anemias: Conventional, Herbal, and Homeopathic Treatments." *Clinical Issues In Perinatal & Women's Health Nursing,* Vol. 3 (1991): 357–63.

Himmelmann, Arnold. "Blood Pressure and Left Ventricular Mass in Children and Adolescents: The Hypertension in Pregnancy Offspring Study." *Blood Pressure.* (October 1994): 1–46.

Hoffman, David. *The New Holistic Herbal.* Rockport, Mass.: Element Books, 1992.

Marti, James. *Alternative Health and Medicine Encyclopedia.* Detroit, Mich.: Gale Research, 1994.

Yee, John D. *Acupuncture in Pain in Infants, Children, and Adolescents.* Baltimore: Williams & Wilkens, 1992.

## CHAPTER 2

### Organizations

American College of Nurse-Midwives. 1522 K Street N.W., Suite 1000, Washington, D.C. 20005.

American College of Obstetricians and Gynecologists (ACOG) Resource Center. 409 12th Street, S.W., Washington, D.C. 20024. Send a brief letter requesting their information on caregiver and birthing options along with a stamped, self-addressed envelope along with the subject of your request.

Doulas of North America (DONA). 110 23rd Avenue East, Seattle, WA 98112.

Informed Birth and Parenting. P.O. Box 3675, Ann Arbor, MI 48106.

International Association of Parents and Professionals for Safe Alternatives in Childbirth. Route 1, Box 646, Marble Hill, MO 63764.

International Childbirth Education Association. P.O. Box 20048; Minneapolis, MN 55420.

Midwives Alliance of North America, founded in 1983, the official registry of midwives in the United States, provides names and telephone numbers of the midwives, and midwife associations in each state. They can be contacted at: P.O. Box 127, Raymond, Ohio 43067. (513) 246-3892. Some states (and provinces in Canada) allow registered midwives who, although not nurses, have passed courses in midwifery.

National Association of Childbirth Assistants (NACA). 205 Copco Lane, San Jose, CA 95123.

National Commission for the Certification of Acupuncturists. 1424 16th Street N.W., Suite 601, Washington, D.C. 20036. (202) 232-1404.

National Women's Health Network. 1325 G Street N.W., Washington, D.C. 20005.

Read Natural Childbirth Foundation. P.O. Box 15056, San Rafael, CA 94915.

### Recommended Reading

Gerber, R. *Vibrational Medicine.* Sante Fe, New Mexico: Bear & Company, 1988.

Goldberg, Burton. *Alternative Medicine: The Definitive Guide.* Payallup, Washington: Future Medicine Publishing, 1993.

Health Insurance Association of America. "The Cost of Maternity Care and Childbirth in the U.S." *Research Bulletin* R15899. December 1989.

Huard, Peter. *Chinese Medicine.* New York: McGraw-Hill, 1968.

Koltyn, Katherine. "Mood Changes in Pregnant Women following an Exercise Session and a Parental Information Session. *Women's Health Issues.* (Winter 1994): 191–95.

Lucas, Vicki. "Birth: Nursing's Role in Today's Choices." *RN.* (June 1993): 38–47.

Murray, Michael, and Pizzorno, Joseph. *Encyclopedia of Natural Medicine.* Rocklin, Calif.: Prima Publishing, 1991.

Simkin, Penny. *The Birth Partner: Everything You Need to Know to Help a Woman Through Childbirth.* Cambridge, Mass.: The Harvard Common Press, 1989.

## CHAPTER 3

### Organizations

Alcoholics Anonymous. Provides pamphlets on alcoholism. 468 Park Avenue South, New York, NY 10016, or check Alcoholics Anonymous listing in your local directory.

American College of Addictionality and Compulsive Disorders. 5990 Bird Road, Miami, FL 33155. (305) 661-3474.

American College of Obstetricians and Gynecologists (ACOG) Resource Center. 409 12th Street, S.W., Washington, D.C. 20024. For a complete list of ACOG pamphlets on nutrition for pregnant and lactating women, send a brief letter with a stamped, self-addressed envelope.

March of Dimes Birth Defects Foundation. "Healthy Eating During Pregnancy." 1275 Mamaroneck Avenue, White Plains, NY 10705. Send SASE for a copy of "Healthy Eating During Pregnancy," which it distributes for the International Food Information Council Foundation.

National Cocaine Hotline. Information and referrals for cocaine users and their families. (800) COCAINE.

National Council on Alcoholism. Provides information and materials. 733 Third Avenue, New York, NY 10017. (800) NCA-CALL, or check your local or state affiliate.

National Institute on Drug Abuse. Information and referrals for drug abusers and their families. (800) 662-HELP.

## Recommended Reading

Balch, James F., and Balch, Phyllis. *Prescription for Nutritional Healing.* Garden City Park, N.Y.: Avery Publishing, 1993.

Braly, James. *Dr. Braly's Diet & Nutrition Revolution.* New Canaan, Conn.: Keats Publishing, 1992.

Editors. "Low-Pressure Pregnancy: Antioxidants And Preeclampsia." *Prevention.* (March 1994): 20–22.

Eisenberg, Arlene. *What to Eat When You're Expecting.* New York: Workman Press, 1986.

Goldberg, Burton. *Alternative Medicine: The Definitive Guide.* Seattle, Wash.: Future Medicine Publishing, 1994.

Hess, Mary, Abbott, Mary, and Hunt, Anne. *Eating for Two: The Complete Guide to Nutrition during Pregnancy.* New York: Macmillan/Collier Publishing, 1992.

Springer, Noel. "Using Early Weight Gain and Other Nutrition-Related Risk Factors to Predict Pregnancy Outcomes." *Journal Of American Dietetics.* (March 1992): 217–19.

Swinney, Bridget. *Eating Expectantly: The Essential Eating Guide and Cookbook for Pregnancy.* Minnetonka, MN: Meadowbrook Press, 1996.

## CHAPTER 4

## Organizations

American College of Obstetricians and Gynecologists (ACOG) Resource Center. 409 12th Street, S.W., Washington, D.C. 20024. For ACOG materials on exercise, send a brief letter along with a stamped, self-addressed envelope.

President's Council on Physical Fitness and Health. 450 Fifth Street N.W., Washington, D.C. 20001.

The American Physical Therapy Association (APTA). P.O. Box 37257, Washington, D.C. 20013.

## Recommended Reading

Nieman, David. *Fitness and Your Health.* Palo Alto, Calif.: Bull Publishing, 1993.

Nieman, David. *Fitness and Sports Medicine: An Introduction.* Palo Alto, Calif.: Bull Publishing, 1992.

Schatz, Mary. *Back Care Basics: A Doctor's Gentle Yoga Program for Back and Neck Pain Relief.* Berkeley, Calif.: Rodmell Press, 1992.

Shapiro, Howard. *The Pregnancy Book for Today's Woman.* New York: HarperCollins, 1993.

Stillerman, Elaine. *Mother Massage: A Handbook for Relieving the Discomforts of Pregnancy.* New York: Delacorte, 1992.

Tapley, Donald. *The Columbia University College of Physicians and Surgeons Complete Guide to Pregnancy.* New York: Columbia University Press, 1988.

## CHAPTER 5

## Organizations

American College of Obstetricians and Gynecologists (ACOG). Send a brief letter requesting ACOG pamphlets on preventing exposure to toxins and stress reduction to: ACOG Resource Center, 409 12th Street S.W., Washington, D.C. 20024–2188.

Consumer Product Safety Commission. 5401 Westbard Avenue, Bethesda, MD 20207.

Environmental Protection Agency (EPA). 401 M Street S.W., Washington, D.C. 20460.

Food and Drug Administration (FDA). 5600 Fishers Lane, Rockville, MD 20857. Provides pamphlets on exposure to food toxins.

Mindfulness Meditation Practice. Box 547, Lexington, MA 01273. Provides Buddhist meditation tapes presented by Dr. Jon Kabat-Zinn, Ph.D., which were developed for the Stress Reduction Clinic at the University of Massachusetts Medical Center.

National Institute for Occupational Safety and Health (NIOSH). 200 Constitution Avenue, Washington, D.C. 20210.

Pace Education Systems (CSM Self-Regulated Course), Inc. Box 113, Kendall Park, NJ 08824. (908) 297-9101. Provides meditation courses, including audiotapes and instruction books on relaxation and stress management.

## Recommended Reading

Federal Drug Administration (FDA). "Lead Threats Lessen, But Mugs Pose Problem." *FDA Consumer.* (August 1993): 1–7.

Gillespie, Clark. *Your Pregnancy: Month by Month.* New York: Harper & Row, 1985.

Pearson, David. *The Natural House Book.* New York: Simon & Schuster, 1989.

Stanway, Andrew. *The Natural Family Doctor.* New York: Simon & Schuster, 1987.

## CHAPTER 6

## Organizations

American Heart Association. 7320 Greenville Avenue, Dallas, TX 75231. For articles on heart disease, high blood pressure, and pregnancy, send self-addressed stamped envelope.

Herpes Resource Center (HRC), American Social Health Association (ASHA). 260 Sheridan Avenue, Palo Alto, CA 94306. Publishes *The Helper,* a quarterly newsletter on treatments for herpes.

National High Blood Pressure Information Center. 4733 Bethesda Avenue, Bethesda, MD 20814.

National VD Hotline. 800-227-8922. Provides information on herpes.

## Recommended Reading

Agras, Winston. "Relaxation Therapy in Hypertension." *Hospital Practice.* (May 1983): 129–37.

Hausman, Patricia. *The Healing Foods: The Ultimate Authority on the Curative Power of Nutrition.* Emmaus, Penn.: Rodale Press, 1989.

Rowan, Robert L. *How to Control High Blood Pressure without Drugs.* New York: Ballantine Books, 1986.

Sarkar, Saul. "Antiviral Effect of the Extract of Culture Medium of Lentinus Edodes Mycelia on the Replication of Herpes Simplex Virus Type 1." *Antiviral Research.* (April 1993): 293–303.

Singh, Raul. "Dietary Modulators of Blood Pressure in Hypertension." *European Journal of Clinical Nutrition.* (1990): 19–32.

## CHAPTER 7

## Organizations

American College of Nurse-Midwives. 1522 K Street N.W., Suite 100, Washington, D.C. 20005.

ASPO/Lamaze. 1200 19th Street N.W., Suite 300, Washington, D.C. 20036–2401. 800-368-4404.

Bradley Classes. American Academy of Husband-Coached Childbirth. P.O. Box 5224, Sherman Oaks, CA 91413. 800-4-BIRTH.

Doulas of North America (DONA). 110 23rd Avenue East, Seattle, Washington 98112.

Informed Birth and Parenting. P.O. Box 3675; Ann Arbor, MI 48106. (313) 662-6857. Distributes *Special Delivery* by Rahima Baldwin, which includes detailed information on pregnancy and birth, finding an attendant, emergency backup, and understanding complications. Also *Pregnant Feelings,* by Rahima Baldwin and Terra Richards, and *Informed Homebirth,* which lists state midwifery organizations.

International Association of Parents and Professionals for Safe Alternatives in Childbirth. Route 1, Box 646, Marble Hill, MO 63764.

International Childbirth Education Association. P.O. Box 20048, Minneapolis, MN 55420.

Read Natural Childbirth Foundation. P.O. Box 150956, San Rafael, CA 94915. (415) 456-8462.

## Recommended Reading

Gach, Michael. *Acu-Face Lift Beauty Workbook.* Berkeley, Calif.: Acupressure Institute, 1994.

Gillespie, Clark. *Your Pregnancy: Month by Month.* New York: Harper & Row, 1985.

Tapley, Donald. *The Columbia University College of Physicians and Surgeons Complete Guide to Pregnancy.* New York: Columbia University Press, 1988.

# Chapter 8

## Organizations

Juvenile Products Manufacturers Association. 236 Route 38 West, Suite 100, Morestown, NJ 08057. Send a self-addressed stamped envelope for *Safe and Sound for Baby,* their free guide on designing your baby's room.

Maternal Fitness. (212) 353-1947. Sells *Coming Contractions: Pain Management for Labor* ($15) by Lulie Tupler, R.N., a very positive videotape which reassures women that labor is natural and not frightening. Details self-hypnosis exercises to use before and during labor.

## Recommended Reading

Hess, Mary, Abbott, Mary, and Hunt, Anne. *Eating For Two: The Complete Guide to Nutrition during Pregnancy.* New York: Macmillan/Collier Publishing, 1992.

Swinney, Bridget. *Eating Expectantly: The Essential Eating Guide and Cookbook for Pregnancy.* Minnetonka, MN: Meadowbrook Press, 1996.

# Chapter 9

## Organizations

American College of Nurse-Midwives. 1522 K Street N.W., Suite 100, Washington, D.C. 20005. Distributes literature on cesareans and VBACs.

American College of Obstetricians and Gynecologists (ACOG). ACOG Resource Center, 409 12th Street S.W., Washington, D.C., 20024–2188. Provides information, statistics, and guidelines for cesareans; also provides pamphlets to help fathers understand the surgical procedure.

ASPO/Lamaze. 1200 19th Street N.W., Suite 300, Washington, D.C. 20036–2401. 800-368-4404. Provides pamphlets on birthing options.

Bradley Classes. American Academy of Husband-Coached Childbirth. P.O. Box 5224, Sherman Oaks, CA 91413. 800-4-BIRTH. Provides literature used in their courses.

Informed Birth and Parenting. P.O. Box 3675, Ann Arbor, MI 48106. (313) 662-6857. Provides *Informed Homebirth,* a twelve-page booklet detailing advantages and disadvantages of home birth.

International Association of Parents and Professionals for Safe Alternatives in Childbirth. Route 1, Box 646, Marble Hill, MO 63764.

International Childbirth Education Association. P.O. Box 20048, Minneapolis, MN 55420.

## Recommended Reading

"Aspirin Offers Hope for Problem Pregnancies." *Prevention.* (May 1996): 54.

Donovan, Bernard. *The Cesarean Birth Experience.* Boston: Beacon Press, 1986.

"Saving Preemies." *Your Health.* (January 11, 1994): 56.

# CHAPTER 10

## Organizations

The American College of Nurse-Midwives. 818 Connecticut Ave. N.W., Suite 900, Washington, D.C. 20006. Send SASE for materials on labor and childbirth and a directory of state nurse midwife organizations.

Informed Birth and Parenting. P.O. Box 3675, Ann Arbor, MI 48106. (313) 662-6857. Call for materials on labor exercises. They also sell *Five Women/Five Births,* a video by Suzanne Arnold that features two births at home—a cesarean, vaginal breech, and a birth-center birth.

## Recommended Reading

Jordan, Sandra. *Yoga for Pregnancy.* New York: St. Martin's Press, 1987.

Tapley, Donald. *The Columbia University College of Physicians and Surgeons Complete Guide to Pregnancy.* New York: Columbia University Press, 1988.

Tracher, Gayle. *An Easier Childbirth: A Mother's Workbook for Health and Emotional Well-being during Pregnancy and Delivery.* New York: Tarcher, 1991.

# CHAPTER 11

## Organizations

American College of Nurse-Midwives. 1522 K Street N.W., Suite 1000, Washington, D.C. 20005.

American College of Obstetricians and Gynecologists. 409 12th Street S.W., Washington, D.C. 20024.

American Society for Psychoprophylax in Obstetrics/Lamaze. 1840 Wilson Boulevard, Suite 204, Arlington, VA 22201.

Informed Birth and Parenting. P.O. Box 3675, Ann Arbor, MI 48106. (313) 662-6857.

International Association of Parents and Professionals for Safe Alternatives in Childbirth. Route 1, Box 646, Marble Hill, MO 63764.

International Childbirth Education Association. P.O. Box 20048, Minneapolis, MN 55420.

Read Natural Childbirth Foundation. P.O. Box 15056, San Rafael, CA 94915.

## Recommended Reading

Auckett, Amelia. *Baby Massage.* New York: Newmarket Press, 1982.

Cox, Connie. *Maternity Massage.* New York: Stress Less Publishing, 1994.

Stillerman, Elaine. *Mother Massage.* New York: Dell Publishing, 1992.

# CHAPTER 12

## Organizations

American College of Obstetricians and Gynecologists. 409 12th St. S.W., Washington, D.C. 20024. Send SASE for materials on postpartum exercises, nutrition, and baby care.

American Sudden Infant Death Syndrome Institute. 275 Carpenter Drive, Atlanta, GA 30328.

International Association of Infant Massage Instructors (IAIMI). Sells *Nurturing Touch Instruction,* a sixty-minute video by Kalena Babeshoff, President of IAIMI. (202) 857-1128.

La Leche League International. 1400 N. Meacham Road, Schaumburg, IL 60173–4840. La Leche League offers information on breastfeeding primarily through personal help.

Call 800-LA-LECHE for toll-free counseling or check your local telephone directory.

National Sudden Infant Death Foundation. 8200 Professional Place, Suite 104, Landover, MD 20784.

## Recommended Reading

American College of Obstetricians and Gynecologists (ACOG). "Diagnosis and Management of Postpartum Hemorrhage." *ACOG Technical Bulletin No. 143,* July 1990.

Bing, Elisabeth. *Losing Weight After Pregnancy: A Step-by-Step Guide to Postpartum Fitness.* New York: Hyperion, 1994.

Brazelton, T. Berry. *What Every Baby Knows.* New York: Delta/Seymour Lawrence, 1983.

Briggs, Gerald. *Drugs in Pregnancy and Lactation: A Reference Guide to Fetal and Neonatal Risk.* Baltimore: Williams & Wilkins, 1994.

Hilchey, Tim. "New Drug May Prevent Jaundice in Newborns." *New York Times.* (January 18, 1994): B6.

Krampf, Leslie. "Baby Your Baby's Skin." *Delicious.* (September 1996): 55.

Sapsted, Anne-Marie. *Banish Post-Baby Blues.* Wellingborough, England: Thorsons Publishing Group, 1990.

Sears, William M. *The Birth Book.* New York: Little, Brown & Company, 1994.

Swinney, Bridget. *Eating Expectantly: The Essential Eating Guide and Cookbook for Pregnancy.* Minnetonka, MN: Meadowbrook Press, 1996.

# $\mathscr{A}$PPENDIX D:
# RECOMMENDED DIETARY ALLOWANCES

| CATEGORY | | PROTEIN (g) | FAT-SOLUBLE VITAMINS | | | |
|---|---|---|---|---|---|---|
| | | | Vitamin A (µg RE)[A] | Vitamin D (µg) | Vitamin E (mg)[B] | Vitamin K (µg) |
| Pregnant | | 60 | 800 | 10 | 10 | 65 |
| Lactating | 1st 6 months | 65 | 1,300 | 10 | 12 | 65 |
| | 2nd 6 months | 62 | 1,200 | 10 | 11 | 65 |

| CATEGORY | | WATER-SOLUBLE VITAMINS | | | | | | |
|---|---|---|---|---|---|---|---|---|
| | | Vitamin C (mg) | Thiamine (mg) | Riboflavin (mg) | Niacin (mg NE)[C] | Vitamin $B_6$ (mg) | Folate (µg) | Vitamin $B_{12}$ (µg) |
| Pregnant | | 70 | 1.5 | 1.6 | 17 | 2.2 | 400 | 2.2 |
| Lactating | 1st 6 months | 95 | 1.6 | 1.8 | 20 | 2.1 | 280 | 2.6 |
| | 2nd 6 months | 90 | 1.6 | 1.7 | 20 | 2.1 | 260 | 2.6 |

| CATEGORY | | MINERALS | | | | | | |
|---|---|---|---|---|---|---|---|---|
| | | Calcium (mg) | Phosphorus (mg) | Magnesium (mg) | Iron (mg) | Zinc (mg) | Iodine (µg) | Selenium (µg) |
| Pregnant | | 1,200 | 1,200 | 300 | 30 | 15 | 175 | 65 |
| Lactating | 1st 6 months | 1,200 | 1,200 | 355 | 15 | 19 | 200 | 75 |
| | 2nd 6 months | 1,200 | 1,200 | 340 | 15 | 16 | 200 | 75 |

[A] Retinol equivalents. 1 retinol equivalent = 1 µg retinol or 6 µg β-carotene. See text for calculation of vitamin A activity of diets as retinol equivalents. As cholecalciferol. 10 µg cholecalciferol = 400 IU of vitamin D.

[B] χ–Tocopherol equivalents. 1 mg d-α tocopherol = 1 α-TE. See text for variation in allowances and calculation of vitamin E activity of the diet as tocopherol equivalents.

[C] NE (niacin equivalent) is equal to 1 mg of niacin or 60 mg of dietary tryptophan.

*Adapted from* J. Marti, *The Ultimate Consumer's Guide to Diets and Nutrition.* Boston: Houghton Mifflin, Inc.;1997: pp. 26–7.

# $\mathcal{J}$NDEX